Juice Fasting Simplified, a Practical Approach

James C. Tibbetts, MBA

ISBN: 978-1-329-17362-0

Disclaimer Notice: You have the constitutional right to prescribe for yourself and to determine your own diet and detoxification methods but the writers and publisher assume no responsibility. If you use the information in this book without the approval of a health professional, you prescribe for yourself, which remains your constitutional right. In addition while it would be inappropriate for the authors to steer individuals in decisions of omission or commission regarding therapies, it would be equally improper to shun responsibility of suggesting what we consider the best options for degenerative disease. The authors and publisher do not directly or indirectly dispense medical advice or prescribe the use of fasting or diet or other modality as a form of treatment for sickness without medical approval. Nutritionists and other health experts in the field of health and nutrition hold widely varying views. The authors and publisher do not intend to diagnose or prescribe.

The Scripture citations are taken in part or whole from various bibles including: *The New American Bible* (Thomas Nelson Publisher, 1970); *The Jerusalem Bible* (Doubleday & Co., 1966); *Revised Standard Version, Holy Bible from the Ancient Eastern Text*, translation from the *Aramaic of the Peshitta* by George M. Lamsa, (Harper San Francisco,1961).

Originally published as *Juice Fasting a Scientific, Practical Approach* (2003, 2008).

Jim Tibbetts
P.O. Box 2533
Glenville, NY 12325

www.jimtibbetts.com

ISBN: 978-1-329-17362-0

Table of Contents

Introduction

Jim Tibbetts has been fasting since 1980 with both short fasts and longer fasts which he does at least once a year. He has done over forty seven day fasts or longer fast (mostly juice and some water) including 14, 21 day fasts and two 40 day juice fasts.

This book is a revision of: *Juice Fasting a Scientific and Practical Approach*, (2003). This earlier work was much longer with more historical material and sections for longer fasts, testimonials. Jim's testimonials of his fasting were deleted and a new book was made: *A Diary on Juice Fasting*, which is a dairy on many of Jim's long fasts.

The author Jim has been looking into the diets of Jesus and Mary since the 1980's and after extensive research his first book on fasting was on *Biblical Fasting* (1998), later he published the books: *Biblical Nutrition the Kosher Vegetarianism of Jesus and Judaism* (2003); *Biblical Nutrition Forty Days of Meditations* (2004); *Biblical Nutrition & Fasting* (2008) and *Jesus and Mary were Kosher Vegetarians, the Evidence from the Bible, the Early Church and Nutrition* (2014).

This book explains the two basic types of fasting: water fasting and juice. It also explains the basic lengths of fasting: three day fast, seven to ten day fasts and longer 14 to 28 day fasts. It goes over various techniques and methods of fasting and various professional opinions on fasting.

The purpose of this work is three fold.
- First it is to give a basic scientific approach using some of the leading experts and research in the field, as well as my own insights.

- Second is to give a practical approach that most anyone can use to guide themselves on a fast under ten days or even 14 to 21 days.
- Third is to give some Therapeutic Fasting understanding and evidence.

This book is trying to give a straight forward, practical, do-it-yourself guide on fasting with everything a person needs for a fast between one and ten days or to go beyond it to 21 days. Hopefully this book will give people some solid knowledge on the topic and to help people develop their discipline on fasting and their own Personal Fasting Program.

Fasting is a main discipline in most religions and it is also a penitential or purification activity in Christian churches, especially in the Catholic and Orthodox Church. Fasting means or implies purification; it is a major means of purification for the body and for the soul.

Fasting is something that needs to become a way of life to achieve its full benefit from doing both short fasts and longer fasts. Hopefully this book will help you in your quest for superior health: in your physical body, your soul (psychological) and your human spirit. Through this you might live a long life of health, happiness and holiness.

Thank you for your interest. Peace to you.

For your health and healing

Jim Tibbetts

I. The Science of Fasting

1. The Physiology of Fasting

"Whatever you eat, whatever you drink, whatever you do at all, do it for the glory of God." 1 Cor 11.31

The food we eat goes through several stages; first it is chewed, masticated; then digested and assimilated; and finally eliminated as waste. The four main organs of elimination are the bowels, the kidneys, the lungs and the skin. A meal goes from the mouth through a thirty-foot tube known as the gastrointestinal tract to the rectum. Liquid passes through about two million filtering fibers in the human kidneys. The body with all its organs, works harmoniously through these stages to bring nutrition to the billions of body cells.

The bowels eliminate two things; food wastes and body waste. Food waste is from the food we eat. The body waste is from the blood and tissues which are discharged into the intestinal canal and in the bowels, these body wastes are excreted from the body. If the body waste is not eliminated, it would cause protein petrifaction resulting in toxemia or acidosis. The kidneys excrete the end products of food and body metabolism from the liver. Perspiration throws off toxins through the sweat glands. The lungs give off carbon dioxide and possibly other gases. This internal elimination is accelerated during the fasting process.

The process of autolysis or self-digestion occurs during a fast. During the first few days, the body will live on its own fast and stored substances. After this is depleted, the body starts to burn and digest its own tissues. The body first burns up the cells which are dead, aged, damaged and

1

diseased tissues, tumors, fat deposits, etc. Fasting gets rid of the inferior cells and keeps the essential ones.

Fasting is not starving. Starving is the process of dying. When a person does not eat, the body enters into a fasting period. This second period can go on for weeks or even a month or two. This third period that a person's body enters into is the stage of starvation. The fasting stage continues as long as the body has stored reserves in the tissues. During this fasting stage, the body continues to nourish itself just as if it were eating. And detoxification also occurs at this time.

When the fasting stage is over with, genuine hunger is experienced. The hunger pains in the beginning of a fast are normal gastric contractions or stomach spasms. These are merely the sensation of hunger and not true hunger. This false hunger is normal for the first few days of a fast.

The body suppresses appetite through a compound called ketones. Ketones are the broken down products of fatty acids. There is an increase in the output of ketones when a person is fasting. These ketones are released into the bloodstream. The appetite is suppressed as there is an increase in the amount of ketones. The fast must be broken when the appetite returns. Fasting can help restore the acid-alkaline balance in the blood. The bloodstream should be alkaline.

During a fast there may be some aches and pains and general discomfort of certain times during the fast. Headaches, sleeplessness, a slight depression, and other minor crises just represent part of the cleansing process. The liver may work overtime putting bile into the stomach causing nausea and vomiting. (If the vomiting continues, perhaps the fast should be broken.) The heart, circulation and respiration may slow down giving a feeling of weakness. As the cleansing process continues, the vigor will return.

The cells in our body exist in three stages; new developing cells, fully developed cells and old dying cells needing to be replaced. Waste products in the cells interfere with the nourishment of the cells. These older dying cells and poisoned cells need to be flushed out of our bodies. *By fasting, these cells with the mucus, toxins and poisons will be flushed out of the body through the kidneys.*

There are more than 200 different cell types and there are about 50-100 trillion cells in the entire body. As cells die or are destroyed, new ones are formed, so the numbers of cells within each body are constantly changing. It is estimated that half of our cells are working in peak condition, one-fourth are in the process of growth, and one fourth are in the process of dying and replacement.

Most advocates of fasting believe that one cause of disease is toxin saturation at the cellular level. Every cellular function produces toxic waste products and fasting helps get rid of these cells or there wastes. Another benefit is that the immune system's workload is greatly reduced during fasting because the digestive tract is spared of any inflammation due to food allergic reactions from processed food, sugars, grains and proteins. Furthermore, the serum fats in the blood are also reduced. This thins the blood and allows more oxygen to get to the tissues.

There are toxins and poisons stored in the fat tissues, such as pesticides and other chemicals which are mobilized and released from the system. Because toxic waste products interfere with the functioning of the cell, it is important that toxins, poisons, diseased and dying cells are eliminated from the system as efficiently as possible. This elimination stimulates the growth of more functional cells. Fasting triggers a cleansing process that affects every cell and tissue in the body. It eliminates dead, diseased and dying cells while stimulating generation of new cells. During a fast, toxic waste products that impair nourishment of cells are eliminated with restoration of normal metabolic rates and higher oxygenation of cells.

Animals when sick or wounded abstain from foods and fast, this is their instinctive way. Man is the only animal that eats when he is sick. Yet, animals do not have religion and fasting usually comes out of strong religious traditions with many good habits. The Tradition of Lent is one habit, among Catholics and Orthodox. Lent occurs at the end of the winter which is a good time to fast and back off from eating a lot and clean house, physically, mentally and spiritually.

Fasting is part of Nature's laws of self-healing and restoration. The absence of food sets the cleansing process in motion. The overburdened organism from its high intake of unusable food is allowed to relax and excessive pressure is relieved. The mucus which lines the inner walls causing obstruction is washed out. Poisonous substances are dissolved and eliminated. The whole body is rejuvenated through the strengthening and purifying power of the fast.

A lot of diseases and physical problems did not exist two hundred years ago before the industrial age. Unfortunately on a global scale we are weakening our immune system generation after generation. For example most of the foods eaten today are full of sugar. Sugar turns to alcohol and stimulates the brain, liver and other organs.

Fasting does two main things: it detoxifies the body and it resets the biochemistry of the body back to its normal operating levels and functional settings (i.e. pH levels). The previous abnormal, messed up biochemistry becomes normal and functionally correct.

Fasting and Addictions

Another aspect of the physiology of fasting is that it can be effective in breaking addictions.

Fasting and prayer can help to break addictions. Addiction is anything that controls a person, whether it's food, TV, pornography, coffee, or drugs; the result is the same. Addiction destroys health and freedom. The food industry has mastered addictive foods by adding lots of salt, fats, processed sugar and artificial flavor enhancers. Once in the blood, what seems to be a delicious treat becomes tomorrow's craving. These daily cravings become powerful forces shaping our destiny through dictating our thoughts, emotions and will. Living becomes a daily routine of subconscious patterns. If we study the patterns, we can discover the triggers for different subconscious actions and desires; such as feeling bad can trigger the urge for junk food. These little prods of addiction keep us in the same routine day after day.

We live in an addictive society where it is socially acceptable to be addicted to sugar, salt, caffeine, fried food, cookies, cakes and junk. An addiction makes you feel good for a time, but, behind your back, it is stealing your self-control and making you its slave through the desire for more. *...for a man is a slave to whatever has mastered him.*" (2 Pet 2:18,19) Fasting, especially the longer seven day fasts, can be helpful with addictions.

2. What Poisons and Toxins in my Body?

Today in the area of nutrition,
"My people are being destroyed from lack of knowledge."
Hos 4:6

During fasting the process of detoxification occurs and poisons and toxins are released from the body. Obviously the next question is what poisons and toxins in my body?

Many books have been written to answer that question. Today there are many chemicals that have toxic effects on the body. These can come from prescription drugs, cleaning compounds, kitchen detergents, garden insecticides and industrial chemicals. A few of the common poisons are: Carbon monoxide from air pollution; DDT and other pesticides sprayed on foods; mercury; lead from gasoline, paint and other industrial sources; ozone, nitrogen dioxide and cadmium are air pollutants coming from smog; wax sprayed on fruits and vegetables to give a longer shelf life and makes them look better; most food colorings are synthetic and coal-tar based; artificial flavorings are either natural or synthetic and comprise about two thirds of all food additives used in America. And irradiation kills the enzymes not just bacteria and germs.

Examples of unnatural chemicals found in the house could be: Arsenic in bug killer; Antimony in eye liner; Barium in lipstick; Cobalt in laundry and dishwater detergent; Copper in water from old metal pipes; Titanium in metal dental ware; Lead in solder in copper pipe joints; Chromium in eyebrow pencils and water softener salts; Vanadium in diesel fuel, candles; Nickel in metal jewelry, metal glasses, watch bands and tooth fillings; Freon in refrigerators, air conditioners and spray cans; Mercy and Thallium in cotton balls, sanitary napkins; Dysprosium in paint and varnish; Holmium in hand cleaners; Hafnium in nail polish and hair spray; Bismuth in cologne; Cesium in clear glass plastic; Tin and Strontium in toothpaste; Erbium in foil packaging; Radon in crawlspaces under the house; Anthanum in copier ink; Aluminum in salt, cans, lotions; Tungsten in electric frying pans, hair curlers, toasters and tea kettles; Beryllium in lawn mowers and kerosene; Formaldehyde in foam mattresses, new clothing, foam chairs.

Both domestic and imported produce is monitored by the FDA, the best they can. In 1991, the FDA reported these results from its testing of domestic and imported produce:

	Domestic Produce	Imported Produce
Samples tested:	8,281	9,933
No residues found:	64.4%	69.2%
Residues below permitted levels:	34.8%	28.5%
Residues in violation:	0.8%	2.3%

The samples with higher residues in violation are held back, when caught. What is more important than the residues in violation is the addition of this plus the low levels gives a total of domestic produce 35.6% and imported 30.8%. Thus between 30 to 36% of produce has some level of pesticide residues in it. That means one third of the supermarket fruits and vegetables have some kind of pesticides. Hopefully most of these will get flushed out of the body but what about the rest that gets lodged in the cells somewhere in the body?

Fasting is one of the best ways to get rid of poisons, toxins, pesticides, waxes and other synthetic chemicals that can be found in fruits and vegetables. Fasting catabolizes the dead, diseased and pesticide ridden cells and flushes them out of the body. Fasting is the best way to get rid of pesticides.

The FDA (Food and Drug Administration) is understaffed and overworked. They are a government agency created to protect the public in foods, drugs and cosmetics. They have the manpower to inspect only a very small percentage of interstate fruits and vegetables and

7

perhaps one quarter or more of the food processors. The agency daily receives applications for approval, testing and modification of drugs. The processing of each application takes months of work involving FDA members and outside consultants. And unfortunately many of the consumer and health groups have their own agenda. The World Health Organization has ranked the U.S. twelfth in general health.

Yet there is a simple and universal answer to this major worldwide problem. The answer is fasting! Fasting is one of the best methods of ridding the body of commercial poisons and toxins. Fasting is a simple, inexpensive way to insure health and happiness.

Numerous scientific studies have been done showing the chemicals and poisons in the food chain. "During the past three decades, surveillance of toxic exposure in the U.S. population has been a routine governmental practice. Since 1970, for example, the U.S. Environmental Protection Agency (EPA) has conducted the National Human Adipose Tissue Survey (NHATS) to determine the prevalence of fat-soluble toxins in the fat cells in U.S. citizens.[1] The 1986 version of this survey, for example, analyzed 671 adipose tissue specimens to determine the prevalence of 111 toxic compounds."[2]

Studies on tissues and body fluids and bone show the presence of numerous toxins in the body, including toxins that could be in the food or the environment: DDE & DDT &, B-BHC,[3] TCDD,[4] p-DCB,[5] Lead,[6] Mercury,[7] Cadmium,[8] PBBs,[9] 2,5-DCP & l-naphthol & 3,5,6-TCP & 2-naphthol & 3,5,6-TCP & PCP, 4-nitrophenol, (pesticide residues in urine in adults in U.S.)[10] Styrene & Vinyl chloride (packaging migrant), [11] Toluene (Solvent), [12] Xylene (solvent) [13].

And there are also toxins directly related to or in the foods: Acetone (pesticide solvent),[14] Arsenic (arsenical pesticides),[15] Benzene (solvent for pesticide formulations), [16]

Bromobenzene (fumigant precursor),[17] Carbon tetrachloride (former fumigant),[18] Ethylene dibromide (fumigant),[19] Ethylene dichloride (fumigant),[20] Hexane (solvent),[21] Kepone (pesticide),[22] Methoxychlor (insecticide),[23] Methy isobutyl ketone (synthetic flavoring),[24] Methylene chloride (decaffeinator),[25] and studies on coal tar dye colorings containing polycyclic aromatic hydrocarbons.[26]

The use of chemicals in foods has soared from 419 million pounds in 1955 to more than 800 million today. Each of us eats more than three pounds of food additives a year.[27] Added to the intentional and unintentional chemicals in our foods are the chemicals we ingest as medicines. Americans are the most medicated people in the world. Every year we swallow 37 billion doses of therapeutic pills, powders, capsules, and elixirs.[28] No one knows what effect the combinations of pesticides, food additives; and medicines may have.

In addition to the foods we eat and the medicines we take, we fill the sky with 130 tons of noxious chemicals... carbon monoxides, hydrocarbons, nitrogen oxides, sulfur oxides, and particulates. Persons living in New York may inhale the equivalent of 730 pounds of chemicals a year. Just think you astronauts are the average America who have all these poisons and chemicals in you bodies! You need to eat raw living foods and go on a long fast and get rid of all this garbage.

Most medical professionals and scientists don't think in terms of poisons, toxins, pollutants and parasites but the best way to deal with these is fasting. What is the difference between poisons and toxins? Poisons generally come from outside the body as just described above. Toxins are produced from within the body by various means.

Dr. Gabriel Cousens points out that: "A typical modern-day meal featuring a main course of beef, poultry, or fish may contain up to 750 million pathogenic microorganisms per servings, compared to a typical vegan meal containing only 500 pathogenic microorganisms per meal."[29]   So the problem is not just inorganic poisons and pollutants but also living bad microorganisms.

The homeostasis of the body seeks a 7.4 pH and other constant conditions such as a body temperature of 98.6 degrees F, certain glucose levels in the blood, certain amounts of body fluids etc. A major example of the importance of a balance pH is given by Dr. Sherry Rogers, she discusses how cancer cells become like yeast cells with a low pH (very acidic); "The normal pH of a cancer cell is 6.5, while a normal cell is 7.4. As soon as the pH of a cancer cell reaches 7.0, it stops growing; a little higher and it starts dying."[30]

A Dr. Theodore A. Baroody, N.D., D.C., Ph.D. points out, that: "Unfortunately, waste acids that are not eliminated when they should be are reabsorbed from the colon into the liver and put back into general circulation. They then deposit in the tissues. It is these tissue residues that determine sickness or health! Discover what tissue acid wastes are present and begin the process of alkalizing yourself, thus ridding them from the body – the result being superior health, energy and strength to enjoy life fully. He further points out, "To replenish and sustain your alkaline reserves, follow the Rule of 80/20 – which means to eat 80% of your foods from the alkaline-forming list and 20% from the acid-forming list. Research, clinical experience, and the knowledge of the 'greats' in nutrition, have re-confirmed this ideal ratio of 80/20%."[31] Yet, he indicates that 99.85% of the people should have this ratio but people in extremely hot places like the Sahara desert may need a more alkaline-forming diet and people in the North or South Pole may require a more acid forming diet in the long winters.

Dr. Robert Young PhD. D.Sc, a leading expert on pH, explains pH in the role of health and healing. "Most people today understand environmental pollution and how it sickens

10

the Earth: we live off the planet and pollute it with waste. Well, illness is basically the same thing. These morbidly evolved organisms are literally eating us alive and polluting us. The thing is, we pollute ourselves first, thus creating the one physiological disease: pH imbalance/toxicity in our terrain. Toxins and an acid-forming diet disrupt body chemistry, and this loss of balance (i.e., dis-ease) in turn disturbs the central balance of the microzyma. Nutritional deficiencies can have the same effect, but can also be created by acidification: the evolution of microzymas is into bacteria and ultimately into a yeast and fungus Y/F infestation. Y/F can infest the blood and any cell or tissue, causing different symptoms.

As more acid wastes back up and the body slowly stews in its own poisonous wastes, the acid begins to corrode veins, arteries, cells and tissues, leading to high valence cellular disorganization, which the medical community refers to as degenerative disease."[32] "Normal body function and health require adequate alkaline reserves as well as the correct pH in tissues and blood. A major means of ensuring these conditions is the proper dietary ratio of alkaline to acid foods. A ratio of at least 80% to 20% - four parts alkaline to one part acid - is required (possibly 3 to 1 for a healthy person). When the proper ratio is maintained, morbid microforms are discouraged."[33]

If this goes on in everyone what can we do about it? Start doing seven to ten day fasts and go on a raw vegan diet to alkalize yourself and get rid of toxins and poisons in the body!

3. Summary of Some Reasons for Fasting

1. Fasting burns up all the diseased, dying and deal cells and inferior protein and fat tissues.
2. Fasting is a quick way to lose weight.
3. Fasting will lead to a more disciplined diet and habits.
4. Fasting helps with anxiety over not eating.
5. Fasting tones up the flesh to make you look younger.
6. Fasting is perhaps the best method of cleansing the body.
7. Fasting can help build up the body's natural resources and the immune system.
8. Fasting can help reduce high blood pressure and high cholesterol levels and imbalanced pH levels.
9. Fasting can help prevent birth defects and reduce morning sickness.
10. Fasting is a way to rid the body of poisons in the world.
11. Fasting can help clean out the toxins of air pollution.
12. Fasting is good to build endurance and for athletes.
13. Fasting can be used to treat physical illness.
14. Fasting can be used to treat mental illnesses.
15. Fasting can help break bad habits like smoking or drinking alcohol, soda or other addicting beverage.
16. Fasting and prayer can help cast out an evil spirit.
17. Fasting is found in all the world's religions and many also in man great leaders and teachers.
18. Fasting is encouraged in the Bible.
19. Fasting is a requirement by Catholics and Orthodox.
20. Fasting can be a silent protest and help identify with world hunger and the global community.
21. Fasting can help identify with the poor and needy.
22. Fasting can help reduce the desires of the flesh.
23. Fasting is an aid to humility.
24. Fasting can help people live longer.
25. Fasting can help us to be clean inside.

Clean inside means eating foods which flow through us, leaving their amino acid proteins, enzymes, minerals, vitamins, and other vital energies. This food should not stop to putrefy and ferment. Clean inside means having a good acid-alkaline balance in the digestive system, a balance which avoids acid-caused toxic conditions throughout the body. Clean inside means a well-working bloodstream will supplied with health promoting minerals and having a liver capable of detoxifying the impurities which run through it.

Furthermore, there are reasons for our ill health and that we are toxic; 1. environmental poisons and toxins and drugs (coming from outside in);   2. toxins built up within out body on a cellular level (toxins being created on the inside); and 3. parasites and worms within us, (which also give off toxic wastes). Parasites and worms often get within us through eating uncooked food products and many other ways. Fasting may not kill all of them.

One of the primary reasons for doing colonic's is to get rid of parasites and worms. When I went on an 8 day fast I did colonic's and a three inch worm came out of me! Where did it come from, I don't know maybe from one of the many fruits or veggie's that I ate. Studies have shown that at least 15% of everyone in America has parasites and worms, experts say its closer to 30%. Colon therapists who make a living doing this say 50 to70% of all their patients who start doing colonic's have a worms and/or parasites. In undeveloped countries it's even higher. Colon therapy is a standard practice in many parts of Europe and in Germany every medical doctor has a colonic's machine in his office.

The primary way we get poisons is from outside the body. The second way of toxicity is from toxins built up within out body on a cellular level. Most people are congested with toxins on a cellular level from cellular wastes. The body is not able to process out cellular wastes so what we're dealing with is something called, intermediate bi-products of cellular metabolism, or cellular wastes. The cells are surrounded by these wastes and have a hard time getting rid of them.

This is the first thing that fasting does is to detoxify each cell and after a group of cells are detoxified and cleansed their biochemistry resets itself back to its normal operating levels. The previous abnormal, messed up biochemistry becomes normal and functionally correct.

"Happy those who hunger and thirst for what is right: they shall be satisfied." Mt 5:6

4. The Physiological Phases of Fasting

"Man does not live by bread alone but on every word that comes from the mouth of God." Mt 4:4

Professor Rosalind Gruben,[1] in an article on "Fasting and Detox Programmes"[34] gives the four stages of fasting as accepted by the International Association of Professional Natural Hygienists who have expertise in fasting.

"The human body is programmed with the ability to elegantly adapt to periods of time without food intake in cases of food scarcity or when injury or sickness naturally necessitates abstinence. Unlike our cultural experience of immediate access to a vast array of foods at any given time of day or night, most animals in the wild never know from where their next meal is coming. Humans, in their natural environment, also survive on unpredictable nutritional sources as can still be observed amongst some other cultures. Were the body unable to adapt to periods of famine the same way that other mammals can, our species would not have survived beyond its most primitive form.

"Once full adaptation into the fasting state has been allowed to run its course, a new level of healing begins to

---

[1] Professor Rozalind Gruben, H.L.C. A.H.S.I., R.S.A., lives in England and is married to Doug Graham, DC an expert in water fasting.

take place. Fasting can allow the body to literally strip itself down on a cellular level and rebuild anew. The intelligence of the human organism is exquisitely demonstrated by the way in which in the fasting state, the body will preserve its vital tissues and organs while selecting unwanted to dispensable tissues for catabolic breakdown. While the vital organs are fiercely guarded, toxic stores and deranged tissues are utilized for fuel.

"As cells are broken down the central nucleus remains constant but the surrounding cytoplasm is catabolized. It is then reconstructed anew. It is this miracle of natural human physiology that gives rise to fasting's well deserved reputation as a rejuvenator. Studies done on individuals who have undergone extensive fasts (longer than 12 days) consistently show their bodies, on a cellular level, to be 10 - 20 years younger than other individuals of their chronological age. It is during longer fasts of over 12 days duration that, as a result of the body utilizing its dispensable tissues for fuel, tumors are autolyzed."[35]

A. Four Phases of Fasting

"According to the findings of the International Association of Professional Natural Hygienists, the following describes the physiological adaptations that the body goes through in order to shift from extrinsic to intrinsic chemical energy reliance.

"Understand that the phases of adaptation are not clear cut in the transitionary process but overlap and "dovetail" to form a smooth physiological shift toward intrinsic independence.

"Phase 1 - This first phase is commonly referred to as the gastrointestinal phase. The body will normally have completed digestive and absorptive tasks 6-8 hours after the last meal is eaten. In instances where the digestive task is much greater, or the digestive abilities compromised, this can take several hours longer. During times of regular alimentation (feeding) it would ten, therefore, be ready for its next "refueling". When further sustenance is not forthcoming, blood glucose levels (BGL) drop. This decrease in available glucose is communicated to the brain which then takes action by initiating phase 2.

"Phase 2 - This is known as the glycolytic phase and occurs 8 - 12 hours after the last meal. recognizing that glucose levels in the blood have taken a dip (by 10% to 20%) the brain instructs the body to liberate glycogen that has been stored in the liver to support the blood sugar. The body can easily accomplish this and the liver glycogen successfully feeds the bloodstream with sugars. The body maintains only a small functional level of glycogen at any given time. A certain amount of it is always reserved to meet the needs of the brain. Because of these two factors, available glycogen soon begins to run low once carbohydrates are no longer ingested. Once again the brain is informed of the need to further support the blood sugar level and responds by initiating phase 3 of the adaptation process.

"Phase 3 - As soon as liver glycogen stores begin to run down the body prepares a "back up" supply of glucose through a process known as gluconeogenesis - literally meaning "the creation of new glucose". In phase 3 muscle protein is broken down to provide glucose. This process is actually set into motion 12 hours after the last meal, and can be evidenced by the fact that urinalysis reveals amino acids to be present in it by morning.

"As was mentioned earlier, the body has the intelligence to be intricately selective in its ability to differentiate between dispensable and indispensable tissues. This is known as the law of selection. In its wisdom, the organism recognizes the need to preserve its lean mass (muscle) and chooses to replace its source of fuel as quickly as possible with expendable, and abundantly available, fat tissue. In 30 - 36 hours following the last intake of food that body will progressively undergo a transition into phase 4, the final state of adaptation in the fast.

"Phase 4 - The catabolism of fat (lipidolysis) provides the body with another alternative way of providing fuel. Due to the prolific availability of fat, even in slender individuals, supplying the body's energy needs this way can continued for an extended period of time. Provision by lipidolysis will continue with re-alimentation (re-feeding) or starvation is allowed to begin.

"Whereas carbohydrates and amino acids provide only 4 calories per gram, fat contains over double that - yielding 9 calories per gram. In a state of complete rest the body requires an average of only 900 calories per day which can be provided by 100 grams of fat. There have been many recorded cases of obese individuals successfully fasting upwards of 120 days by relying on this source of chemical energy.

"As the process of lipidolysis is slightly less efficient than carbohydrate metabolism in providing fuel for muscular contraction, once into Phase 4 individuals commonly experience a slower, although still efficient, mechanical movement.

"The shift of the body's fuel dependence to fat is progressive but will be fully in place, and exclusive to any other form of chemical energy production, 10-12 days into the fast. The body that has a history of fasting experiences may well achieve this soon in 3 - 4 days.

"Similar to the body's ability to cool itself down via the production of sweat, the speed and efficiency which the organism can move through the various stages of fasting adaptation depends on previous demands to do so. The trained endurance athlete has a highly tuned sweat mechanism and is proficient at responding quickly to overheating. The person who has fasted before will find themselves moving more quickly into total fat reliance than a first time faster. Another very influential factor in the speed of transference to fat reliance are the meals taken directly before the onset of the fast."[36]

B. Phases of Fasting and Detox

The Physiological Phases of Fasting can be restated in other terms too. Some fasting experts and scientists often refers to three physiological phases of fasting. The first stage they call the gastro-intestinal phase which includes everything from the mouth to the rectum that processes and digest food. In this phase a person is getting energy for the last meal or two. This is going to last between 6 to 12 hours or more. Then the person has used up most if not all of the fuel from the last meal and they go into the second phase of fasting which is the glycogen phase.

Glycogen is stored up sugar or glucose which is the primary fuel for our body. Glucose is stored mostly in the liver and in the skeletal muscle cells. Our body uses up some reserves of glycogen and this can last a day or two, depending on how much glycogen is stored in the cells of the muscles, liver and elsewhere. But about 50% of the fuel that our muscles are using is coming from fat. This shifts to the phase which is the body burning fat and is called 'fat burning' or 'protein sparing', mode of fasting. The body still needs to consume some glucose and has used some from its reserves.

At this point the body shifts over and starts consuming fat for energy. Here it also first starts getting rid of the fat cells that are dead and diseased and dying. Thus it starts catabolizing the junk fat cells in the body and does house cleaning. In some mysterious way the body has intelligence, an inner consciousness, if you would, and uses this fast to systematically clean house in the body. In this final phase which lasts throughout the 7 to 10 day fast the body catabolizes all the dead and diseased and dying cells. It is this process that often brings healing to the body, or allows the body to heal itself. It is involved in the process of physiological purification in the process of fasting.

During the first stage of the fast, the stomach and digestive tract are emptied and the pH changes to become more alkaline. Weight loss which is mostly water loss is greatest the first few days of the fast. Headaches and hunger pains often occur during the first three days. This first stage is one to three days usually.

Next the intestines and liver start to purge themselves of toxins and poisons; the elimination is mostly through the urine and the skin from the bloodstream. The physiological purgation on this level excretes toxins and poisons trapped in the organs, glands and muscles. Symptoms like a flu may be experienced such as diarrhea, nausea, muscle aches, etc.

In the third stage tissue and cellular cleansing occurs, blood toxins are removed and poisons deeply embedded in the kidneys and intestines are released. The process of catabolism breaks down the diseased and poisoned cells and eliminates them. Usually this third stage has positive emotions connected to it, giving a high or euphoria feeling but there can also be negative feelings as well.

Elimination on the cellular level is important and a long fast helps this to happen. A long fast once or twice a year is needed to keep the body clean at the cellular level. The beneficial effects of a long fast will decrease over time. Six months to a year down the road another long fast will be needed to detoxify the inner body once again.

One thing that happens on the 5th or 6th day often Endorphins (hormones or molecules) get released into the body. These often give a feeling of high or elation on a fast; also if a lot of juice is taken on a fast the fruits can become low levels of alcohol in the body that gives a minor intoxication feeling or high.

C. Confusion with the word Ketosis

Furthermore, when a person is burning fat for energy they are in what is called, ketosis. Ketosis is burning fat for energy and something our body is very good at doing, and is O.K. to do. Sometimes confusion comes about from this word ketosis from two situations: the problem with diabetic's and the activity of high protein meat eating diets.

Ketoacidosis is a problem with diabetic people whose diabetes is not well controlled. Insulin is the key that unlocks the door of the cells and lets glucose into it. But when glucose can't get into the cells the body will shift to using fat. When this happens in a diabetic person they can get high glucose and insulin levels in the blood. The kidneys start letting the glucose out of the body through the bladder and the diabetic gets dehydrated. Ketoacidosis involves these three: high glucose and insulin levels and becoming dehydrated, this is a problem and not healthy. Now ketosis is going on at the same time but this is not the same thing that happens when a person goes on a fast.

The other confusion of ketosis and fasting is with these high protein diets like the Atkins diet which tries to make a person go into ketosis by eating lots of protein. And when the body goes into ketosis the body starts burning fat for energy and the person loses weight. Again this involves a high protein diet and is not the same thing that happens on a fast.

The body needs far less protein during a fast, a normal healthy body only needs 30 to 40 grams of protein a day. During a fast the body needs much less then that probably less than half, or maybe less than a quarter of the protein, studies are unclear on this. But from experience professional fasters know that it is very little. But it is best not to engage in a lot of outer physical activity during a fast, inner mental activity such as reading or writing, meditating or prayer are better. Because by using all the large muscle groups you are creating a demand for glucose.

D. Phases of Liver detox and Free Radicals

Dr. Sherry Rogers in her books goes into detail concerning the phases of detoxification and the liver. There are two phases which the liver uses to detoxify waste products in the blood stream. Phase I is a family of enzymes that are breaking things down and forms different products called 'intermediate metabolites'. Phase II takes these metabolites and uses specific nutrients to get rid of them. Juice fasting does help the nutrient dependency of faze II. For example vitamin C is known to be helpful in the detox process since it often attaches itself to toxins and drags them to the bloodstream to get rid of them. Waste products get defused in the blood stream which gives the kidneys and liver the opportunity to get rid of them.

An additional footnote is that eating produces free radicals and so does fasting and the detoxification process. Juice fasting produces less free radicals then water fasting because juice is nutrient rich and has a lot of anti-oxidants such as vitamin A, C, E, zinc, etc.

Not all free radicals are bad since cells create free radicals to break down destructive toxins. It's only when the free radicals get to parts of the cell that they're not suppose to that these cells can get free radical damage. Fasting has a powerful effect on modulating free radical production, preparing free radical damage and facilitating the removal or detoxification of the products of free radical damage.

This is not to put down water fasting which is a valid way to fast and in some cases might be better then juice fasting. Some water fasting experts say that water fasting is better at releasing more toxins into the body but the scientific evidence may not be available on this debated point. Hey, both work so follow your heart and 'Fast with All Your Heart!'

Alan Goldhamer, D.C. (website) gives a good short explanation of the process of fasting: "The first phase can be called the gastrointestinal phase, and lasts approximately for first six hours following the last meal. During this phase the body uses glucose, amino acids and fats, as they are absorbed from the intestinal tract.

Phase two lasts for more or less the next two days. During this time the body will use its glycogen (sugar) reserves that are stored in the muscle and liver cells. These glycogen reserves are mobilized to provide the central nervous system, including the brain, with its normal fuel, glucose. Within a few hours the body begins to convert adipose (fat) tissue into fatty acids.

Were it not for the body's ability to switch fuels and enter phase three, where the body switches from glucose to fat metabolism, therapeutic fasting could not take place. The body's protein reserves would be quickly depleted."

II. Basic Types of Fasting

1. Water Fasting

"Moreover, when you fast..." Mt 6:16   This is a
direct command to fast, by Jesus.

The three practices that Jesus gives in Matthew 6 are
almsgiving, prayer and fasting. After the Lord 's Prayer
Jesus said, "Moreover, when you fast..." This is an
admonition telling people to fast.

Basically there are two kinds of water; distilled water
and un-distilled water. Un-distilled water is well water,
spring water, lake or river water or sea water. This water has
organic materials in it. Hard water has inorganic minerals in
it. Distilled water is pure water such as rain or snow, yet it is
lacking minerals. Fruit and vegetable juices have natural
sugars, organic minerals and vitamins mixed in with the
distilled water.

There are two sides of the distilled water versus the
mineral water issue. Some claim one is better to drink others
say the other is better. But there is a third view that we
should drink both to balance the acid orientation of distilled
water versus the alkaline orientation of the mineral water.
The pH of distilled water is a bit acidic but this does not
mean we shouldn't drink it. There are reasons to create
acidity or alkalinity.

Dr. Paul Bragg recommends the use of distilled water
on a fast. But Dr. Paavo Airola recommends spring or well
water and does not advise using distilled water. He also
states that the minerals and trace elements in un-distilled
water are beneficial to the body. Dr. Airola also suggests on
tablespoon of pure sea water in a glass of regular water can

be taken each day during a fast. But it is not a big deal; try to drink pure, clean water.

The water molecule (H_20) like other atoms has three degrees of motion. Rotational - moving in a circle, translational - moving in a straight line and vibrational - moving in a vibrating pattern. All water molecules move in these three ways, as well as most all molecules. Thus a molecule can be quicken in its vibrational rate.

Dr. Walker was a leading authority on raw vegetable juices and lived to be 119 years old. He must have been doing something right to live that long. His diet was mostly raw fruits and vegetables. He used to fast only several times a year for three days, with his strict diet, his body was probably so cleansed that he did not need to fast. His book, Raw Vegetable Juices, is a very good book.

N. W. Walker makes a distinction between organic water and inorganic water. Organic water is only found in raw vegetables. Inorganic water is only found in raw vegetable and fruit juices. Inorganic water is from the faucet, rain water, rivers, and streams and from springs. Vegetation changes the inorganic water into the "life-containing atoms of vital organic water." At another place Dr. Walker states, "Natural means to regain and maintain our health at a high rate of vibration...but we deliberately continue into a slow state of toxemic decadence."[37] His insight has scientific potential, but as of yet is debatable.

The body is 70 percent water. To lose a tenth of the water in the human body can be dangerous, to lose a fifth can be fatal. The fluids and cells in the body are all dependent on water. If the human body is deprived of liquids for a few days, it can be fatal. Most foods contain a high percentage of water. Fasting should always be done with liquids, especially water.

Homeostasis of fluids means that the body is in fluid balance. This means that the total amount of water in the body is normal and that it remains relatively constant. It also means relative constancy of the distribution of water in the body's three fluid compartments. The three compartments are the cells, the interstitial spaces (tissue spaces) and in the blood vessels. Fluid imbalance is when both the total volume of water in the body and the amount in one or more of its fluid compartments has increased or decreased beyond its normal limits.

For fasting, a fluid balance is important. Fluid balance if when intake must equal output. Thus if there is a lot of output through urine, sweating, or moisture release through the lungs, then the volume of liquid taken in must equal the volume of liquid leaving.

Water enters the body through three sources: liquids, water in the food and tissue metabolism (water formed in cells when the food is metabolized). Water normally leaves the body by four exits: lungs (water in the expired air), kidney (urine), intestines (feces), and skin (by diffusion and sweat). Thus water intake must equal water output to keep a healthy fluid balance.

Water fasting is the oldest, the most well known and widely used type of fasting. Water fasting is the classic form of fasting. As a science it was popularized in the U.S. around the turn of the century. Obviously fasting on water means drinking only water. There is no set amount as to how much water a person can drink but certainly they should drink more than usual. And drinking a lot of water can offset hunger.

Dr. Bragg recommends an alternative to just drinking water is to add one teaspoon of lemon juice and half a teaspoon of uncooked honey to each glass of water. Make up a quart or two and refrigerate it. By adding these two ingredients, they act as mucus and toxic dissolvers. By dissolving the toxic poisons they can be more easily flushed out through the kidneys. It also helps the water to be more palatable. Adding lemon and honey can be used on a 24-36 hour fast.

Dr. Bragg gives his orientation on fasting, *"Here is my personal fasting program and the one I highly recommend to my students. Every week I take a 24-hour or a 36-hour fast. This I never miss! In addition I fast from seven to ten days, four times a year."*[38]

"After a weekly fast, and four to six fasts of from 3 to 4 days, for about four months, a person would be ready for a seven-day fast. By this time, large amounts of toxic waste have been removed from the body by weekly fasts, the 3- and 4-day fasts, and the good, wholesome, natural diet."[39]

Dr. Bragg states that you should not break a fast with animal products such as meat, milk, cheese, butter, fish, nuts or seeds. Instead break it with a salad and wait until the 2nd meal for animal products. And he suggests that our mind must rule our bodies if we are to fast successfully since 'Flesh is dumb'.

One expert, Linda Page N.D., Ph.D. points out that fluoride is a toxic substance. "Fluoride occurs naturally in some water as calcium fluoride, but most drinking water that contains naturally-occurring fluoride has 0.1 to 0.3 ppm fluoride. The amount usually put into the drinking water is 1.0 ppm. The type of fluoride added to water is a hazardous waste product (hydroflusilicic acid) of the phosphate fertilizer industries. It is an extremely corrosive substance.
"The risks of fluoridating our water supply are significant and the benefits are negligible. Don't forget that our water supply affects our food supply. If you water "organic" vegetables and fruits with fluoridated water, you get fluoride in the produce."[40] A long period of use of chlorinated water has shown a 40% greater chance of bladder cancer.

Fluoride is mandatory in over 60% of the U.S. public drinking water, yet Japan and most of Europe, are 98% fluoridation-free. And there is active opposition in Britain, Australia, and New Zealand as well as in the U.S. Therefore if possible do not use fluoridated water on a fast!

Dr. Page does not recommend long water fasts. "Leading nutritionists and detoxification experts agree that fresh vegetable and fruit juice cleansing is superior to water fasting. Indeed, juice cleansing is an evolution in detoxification methods. Fresh juices, broths and herb teas help deeply cleanse the body, rejuvenate the tissues and guide you to a faster recovery from health problems than water fasting.

"Traditional water fast is harsh and demanding on your body, even in times before huge amounts of food and environmental toxins were part of the picture. Today, it can even be dangerous. Deeply buried pollutants and chemicals from our tissues are released into elimination channels too rapidly during a water fast. Your body is essentially "re-poisoned" as the chemicals move through the bloodstream all at once. Sometimes, the physical and emotional stress of a water fast even overrides the healing benefits.

"Vegetable and fruit juices are alkalizing, so they neutralize uric acid and other inorganic acids, better than water, and increase the healing effects. Juices support better metabolic activity for fasting, too. Metabolic activity slows down during a water fast as the body attempts to conserve dwindling energy resources that further reduce productive cleansing. Juices are very easy on digestion - easily assimilated into the bloodstream. They don't disturb the detoxification process."[41]

Of course Dr. Paul Bragg who has done many long water fasts would disagree with Dr. Linda Page. And there are fasting clinics around the U.S. that only do water fasting. They take people on water fasts for several weeks or more than a month depending on what people need. They have led hundreds of people on long water fasts with great success.

Most experts tend to emphasize one type of fasting over another type of fasting. Some put down one type in favor of another type. Both sides come up with good reasons why their method works the best. For some things water fasting might be better then juice fasting or vice versa. Thus the debate goes on.

My personal opinion (Jim) is that both water fasts and juice fasts are good ways to do fasting. Experts in America tend to use water fasting and experts in Europe tend to emphasize juice fasting. Both work and have helped many people to detox and be healed of many different diseases. Follow your Heart as to what the Lord wants you to do, water or juice fasting.

Whatever type of fasting one goes on the average person has 6 to 8 weeks of reserves in their body before starvation sets in. Juice fasting is definitely easier the water fasting.

Some people feel that they are weak and blame it on the fast but it is usually because of toxins in the body that are being released and dumped into the bloodstream. This also causes lightheadedness. And sometimes people also have an emotional release during a fast. Thus fasting can be healing on an emotional level too.

2. Juice Fasting

"God said, 'See, I give you all the seed-bearing plants that are upon the whole earth, and all the trees with seed-bearing fruit; this shall be your food." Gn 1.29

Juice fasting involves drinking fruit and vegetable juices, vegetables and herbal teas. These are easily assimilated into the upper digestive tract and do not stimulate the secretion of hydrochloric acid in the stomach.

Water fasting has been around for thousands of years whereas juice fasting is mostly found as a practice in this century. The question has been asked if juice fasting is a real fast or just a liquid diet? Dr. Airola responds, "Any condition when your body is encouraged to initiate the process of autolysis, or self-digestion, is fasting. During juice fasting, when no solid foods, proteins or fats are consumed, your body will decompose and burn all the diseased and inferior protein and fat tissues, just as it does during the water fast. Juices are absorbed directly into the bloodstream without the usual process of digestion."[42]

Dr. Airola presents a list of scientific justifications for juice fasting which he bases on physiological facts and professional opinions.
1. Raw Juices and broths "are rich in vitamins, minerals, trace elements and enzymes."
2. "These vital elements are very easily assimilated directly into the bloodstream, without putting a strain on the digestive system - thus they do not disrupt the healing and rejuvenating process of autolysis, or self-digestion."
3. Juices "do not stimulate the secretion of hydrochloric acid in the stomach."
4. "The nutritive elements from the juices are extremely beneficial in normalizing all the body processes, supplying needed elements for the body's own healing

activity and cell regeneration, and, thus, speeding the recovery."

5. "Raw juices and vegetable broths provide an alkaline surplus which is extremely important for the proper acid-alkaline balance in the blood and tissues, since blood and tissues contain large amounts of acids during fasting."

6. "Generous amounts of minerals in the juices, particularly in the vegetable broth, help to restore the biochemical and mineral balance in the tissues and cells."

7. Numerous fasting clinics and experts make scientific claims as well:

a) "According to Dr. Ralph Bircher, raw juices contain an as yet unidentified factor which stimulates what he calls a micro-electric tension in the body and is responsible for the cells' ability to absorb nutrients from the blood stream and effectively excrete metabolic wastes."[43]

b) Dr. Ragnar Berg a leading authority on nutrition and biochemistry states; "During fasting the body burns up and excretes huge amounts of accumulated wastes. We can help this cleansing process by drinking alkaline juices instead of water while fasting. I have supervised may fasts and made extensive tests of fasting patients, and I am convinced that drinking alkaline-forming fruit and vegetable juices, instead of water, during fasting will increase the healing effect of fasting. Elimination of uric acid and other inorganic acids will be accelerated. And sugars in juices will strengthen the heart...Juice fasting is, therefore, the best form of fasting."[44]

c) Dr. Otto H.F. Buchinger at his clinic has supervised over 80,000 fasts and employs only juice fasting. "He told me that, in his experience, fasting on the fresh raw juices of fruits and vegetables, plus vegetable broths and herb teas, results in much faster recover from disease and more effective cleansing and rejuvenation of the tissues that does the traditional water fast."[45]

Drinking juices allows for the body to assimilate all of the vital substances in the quickest possible time. It may only take ten to fifteen minutes to assimilate juices properly made. But it may take several hours to digest juice that is still in the pulp or liquefied stage (with solids). Juices give the cells in the body all the elements they need in a way that is easily assimilated.

Dr. Walker emphasizes that, "During a fast we eat no food whatever. We drink large quantities of water or fruit juices somewhat diluted with water. This dilution is necessary because otherwise the burning up of debris in the system becomes too severe or concentrated. Fruits are the cleansers of the body, and, particularly during a fast, they must be used with discretion, although we may take as much fruit as we want, with benefit, at other times.

The amount of such liquid taken during a fast has usually been not less than 2 quarts, but preferably one gallon or a little more throughout each day of the fast."[46]

Dr. Walker does not believe in long fasts over a week but recommends that people go for 6 or 7 days and then break the fast for 3 or 4 days. For those in need of a prolonged fast he recommends that they do a 6 to 7 day fast break it for 3 or 4 days to get some nutrients in the body and then start the fast up again. This break allows nutrients to restore and build up.

For a seven day fast it takes three days to come off of it correctly. Thus it would probably be better to eat a strict plant-based diet for a week or two and then do another seven day or longer fast.

Even though juice fasting is an excellent way to fast it may not be the best type of fast for everyone. One such problem could be Candia, a yeast problem that exists mostly in women. Candia or yeast is increased by eating sugars and thus the fruit sugar in fruit juice may increase the yeast problem. But fasting could help this problem and even heal the problem. A strict raw veggie diet and juicing could heal the problem. Other conditions could exist that would make water or bread and water fasting a better option. But by taking the right kinds of juices this could be avoided, see Dr. Walker's book on juices.

In addition to much sugar from drinking a juice could deplete minerals, thus add water to juice when drinking large quantities. But for a seven day fast this is not going to be a problem. And when doing a long fast, drinking broths can help replenish the minerals that may be lost. Juice has refined sugar and too much sugar can turn into fat, but for a seven day fast this is not a problem either, since you'll lose weight not gain it.

In a general way it can be said that there are three levels of juices: Juices from the supermarket, juices from the health food store and freshly made juice from a juicer. Most of the juices in the supermarket are not real juices and most are pasteurized above 130 degrees destroying the important vitamins and enzymes. There is little nutrition left in most of these drinks and they are basically sugar flavored water.

The juices in a health food store are usually not killed as much and have some nutrients and good qualities still in them. Health food store juices can sometimes be found in the supermarket in their special health food sections. This is the second level of food value and usable for a long fast.

The third and highest level of juice is made fresh from a juice machine. Juice is always best if you drink it right after you juice it. Oxidation occurs when in contact with air and light or even room temperature. Freshly made juice can easily be stored for one to two days, sometimes three days in a refrigerator. A dark glass jar, such as the prune juice jar is best to store fresh juice. If possible fill the juice to the top to prevent excessive oxidation. Opening and closing the jar will increase the deterioration rate of the juice.

Apple juice and other juices are white or natural colors when first made but with oxidation they will turn brown. Turning brown does not mean that these are bad juices. Bad juice will have a bite or tingle in your mouth, it also may taste sour, smell foul or even coagulate.

Frozen juice and bottled juice are usually pasteurized to some degree which destroys some of the vitamins and enzymes. The process of thawing and freezing in frozen juice is not as bad as pasteurization, canning and irradiation. But it all depends who makes it and the process used. Do not get too hung up on the relative merits of different juices, just realize that there are differences.

Some juices are really not juices from a juicer such as: Apricot, Banana, Blueberry, Cantaloupe, Coconut, Honeydew, Papaya, Peach, and Plum, Prune, Strawberry and others. The pulp does not separate from the liquid in these juices very easily. The pulp is often mixed with water and other operations turn it into a juice. Oftentimes these are mixed with other juices such as apple or orange or grape. Some berries release a little juice but it is mostly a mixture with apple or another juice. There are some fruits like prunes are soaked and then extracting the liquid. Sometimes sweeteners, flavors and color are added.

Fresh juice is usually the best choice for a seven day fast. A long fast just on freshly made juice is a lot of work and expensive, even though health clinics and spas recommend this. Having fresh juice once or twice a day is enough and drink health food store bottled juice the rest of the time. Most juice can be kept for twenty four hours in the refrigerator.

The two juices that are always good to try to make during a long fast are *carrot juice and a green (chlorophyll) juice*. A chlorophyll juice is the 'blood of the plants,' it is the life giving liquid that is the beginning of the food chain and upon which both animal and human life is built. The healing claims of chlorophyll juices and carrot juice are numerous. They both are said to build up and strengthen the tissue cell activity.

One of the reasons that juicing works is because it does not have the pulp which contains mostly fiber and other food materials. The extracted carrot juice has about the same or similar amounts of carotene, vitamin C, potassium and other vitamins and minerals as the pulp of the carrot that is discarded. But the pulp has about six times more fiber and other food materials that make it up.

For a juice fast, like a water fast, you do not want solids put into the stomach which would start the digestion process working.

There are some people who call juice fasting a juice diet. Dr. Joel Robbins DC, MD, promotes a juice diet, which is really a fast, but he allows them to eat a little if it's necessary. He emphasizes that the three main ways to get proper nutrients into the body are: 1. Fresh and Raw Diet; 2. Food Supplements; and 3. Fresh and Raw Juice. The benefits of juicing are many such as getting live nutrition; the juice is easily assimilated; the energy is conserved because of not having to digest the food; the nutrients are concentrated and vitamins and minerals are easily obtained through juicing.

One comment that he makes is worth quoting: "Do not mix fruit juices with vegetable juices. In general, fruits and vegetables are digested utilizing incompatible enzymes in different parts of the digestive tract. Mixing them together can result in a lack of proper digestion along with resulting toxic by-products. If you want to follow a glass of fruit juice by a glass of vegetable juice, provided you are hungry for some more juice, wait at least an hour between glasses." Some exceptions he mentions are that apples do mix well with carrots; celery and lettuce may be juiced with fruit juice; and "Do not mix tomato juice with carrot or potato juice. The acid of the tomato hinders the digestion of the starch in the carrot and potato. All other vegetables mix equally well with either carrot or tomato juice."[47]

3. The Water with Juice Fast

There are two kinds of water fasting: the 'Water Fast' and the 'Water Fast with Juices'. The water fast is nothing but water the whole time while on the fast from beginning to end. You drink as much water as you like all day long.

I (Jim) highly recommend the water fast and in some cases for some people it would be better than doing a juice fast. In the long run juice fasting gets refined and starts becoming closer to a water fast over the years.

Just drinking water can be difficult and it might be best to have two kinds of water available to you. Tap water is usually mineralized, distilled water is not. Having some mineral water and some distilled water available might help the taste buds and allow a subtle variety of switching from one to the other. But just drinking one type of water is fine too.

The 'Water with Juices' can take several forms.

1. It could start with juice and then move to just water and then end with juices. Instead of just drinking water a person could have tea with a little honey.

2. It could start with juice for a day or two and then move to just water and this could have a glass of juice (or water with lemon and honey) a day during the water fast, then break the fast with juices on the last day.

3. A third type would be to have a water fast the whole time with a glass or two of juice and/or water with honey and lemon every day or tea with honey. Then break the fast with juices and food. The famous Paul Bragg ND,

PhD who fasted people for over 70 years[48] used to allow a glass of water with lemon and honey. He said that the lemon and honey also helped to overcome the taste of water, he also said it gave a little extra energy boost and the lemon helped to clean out the intestines.

On all three possibilities of the water fast you would then break the fast with juices and food. The argument against two and three is that these might be called juice fast instead of water fast. But Paul Bragg promoted water fasts using his method and would not consider them a juice fast. Also these are fasts with predominately water whereas a juice fast has predominately juice all day long during the fast.

Water fasting is definitely a more difficult type of fasting and harsher on the body while juice fasting is more gentle. But water fasting does allow quicker weight loss and my go deeper into the tissues which is beneficial for helping the healing process with degenerative diseases.

On a juice fast a person can work a full forty hour week. But to do a water fast and try working full days is too difficult and not a good idea since you will probably have to lay down and rest several times during the day. The fruit sugar in juice fasting gives energy to work from but on a water fast you just do not have that extra energy.

Fasting experts do not recommend trying to work while on a water fast, in fact it would be best to be under supervision and to go to a fasting clinic to do a seven day or longer water fast. Water fasting is much more intense then Juice fasting. As to which is better, water fasting or juice fasting, the debate has been going on for decades and continues among the experts, I think both have value and certain benefits.

A good formula for those just starting out on a water fasting would be to do the second type of water with juices fast. Start the first two days on juices as described in this book. The fast really does not begin until the third day and the first two days is a physiological shift towards fasting. The third day to the six day drink just water with a glass of warm water with lemon and honey during the day if desired. If there's a need a second glass which usually happens with a healing crisis, then have a second glass. Then on the seventh day have a glass of warm water with lemon and honey in the morning. Have a glass of carrot or other juice at lunch and for dinner have another glass of juice. Then the eight day break the fast as described in this book.

The U.S. fasting Institutes tend to emphasize water fasting whereas juice fasting is found more in European health Institutes, both are good. I (Jim Tibbetts) describe both and recommend both, but juice fasting is by far the easiest way to learn and gain experience in fasting. And then a person can gradually move into water fasting.

III. The One to Three Day Juice Fast

1. The One Day Fast

The ancient Jewish people used to fast once or "fast twice a week." Lk 18:12

The one day a week fast is the standard in the world of fasting. I have never read any book on fasting that objects to fasting one day a week. There are two types of fast that can be done for a one day a week fast: the water fast, the juice fast or a possible third is a penitential diet: the bread and water fast.

At first the 24 to 36 hour, one day, weekly fast may be difficult but then it will become a regular part of your weekly schedule. After doing a weekly fast for a year or two, it will become a normal way of life. In fact, you will find it difficult to eat a lot of food if you eat on the day of your weekly fast. The body rhythms and body chemistry, the attitude of the mind and emotions, and the daily life schedule for yourself and others will go much better if you stick to fasting on the same day each week.

Starting a fast in the morning and breaking it the following morning is a normal 24 hour fast. But you can start it at dinner and break it the following dinner. Or for a 36 hour fast start it after dinner and go through the whole next day fasting and then end the following morning. Breakfast means "break a fast" so breaking a fast in the morning is normal and natural.

After several years fasting becomes a habit, a way of life. If you eat on the day that you normally fast you may fill up and would not feel like eating a lot. If you skip a fast for a week or two your body could start desiring to fast, just like it would desire food. Habits become ingrained in us.

At times I've had a juice party and had different exotic juices. Other times juice might not be appealing to me and I would go for water with some lemon and honey, or just plain water.

Then there have been days that I (Jim) went through the school of hard knocks. Once, I was over at my folk's house and my mother had cooked a big meal, after I told her that I had fasted that day, she insisted that I sit down and have a big meal since my body needs the food. So I sat down and ate the big meal she served me. It tasted good but within minutes afterwards, I walked over the sink and threw it up.

One of the first rules on breaking a fast is, do not eat a large meal after a fast! The stomach and intestines have shrunk up a little and cannot accept a lot of food. This is also much more important on longer fasts. One good way to break a 24 hour fast is to have an appetizer an hour or so before eating a small meal. Putting something in the stomach before the meal would start the gastric acid secretions in the stomach, preparing it for a larger meal.

The more a person does a weekly fast the easier it will become. Perhaps starting out fasting a whole day may be too much, all at once. Skip one meal for a month, then skip two meals for a month, then try a 24-hour juice fast. Then after a couple of months of juice fasting try a water fast or try a 36 hour fast. If the one day fast is new or not going well try to hang in there until 3:00 o'clock as a penance since the three o'clock is often associated with the passion.

There are three basic ways to do a 24 hour fast: first is to fast water, the second is to fast on fruit and vegetable juices and the third is juice and water. Fasting one day a week helps to strengthen and purify the body. A weekly one-day fast makes 52 days of body purification a year.

2. The Three Day Fast

A three day fast is an extension of a one day fast, but the fasting process of catabolism starts during the second day so a three day fast is really the first day of a physiological cleansing fast, and you might as well go seven days on the fast.

The three day fast can be more difficult than a seven day fast because it often takes two to three days to get over the hunger sensation. After the second or third day on a seven day fast there are no or few hunger pains. So by the time you are over the hunger sensations on a three day fast you break the fast. The three day fast may be good for some people and circumstances.

Personally I do not recommend a three day fast, because the process of catabolism has just started on the third day and then you stop the fast. If you're going to do a three day fast you might as well push on and do a seven day fast which will give you the most benefit. And the first three days are the most difficult part of a seven day fast. Three day fasts might be beneficial for some types of chronic illness or diseases, so there could be some usage for a three day fast.

Yet scripture does give example of three day fasts:
"When they have all, as one man, obeyed his instructions and had made their petitions to the merciful Lord, weeping, fasting and prostrating themselves for three days continuously..." 2 Mac 13:12

"Go and assemble all the Jews now in Susa and fast for me. Do not eat or drink day or night for three days. For my part, I and my maids will keep the same fast." Est 4:16

"For three days he (Paul) was without his sight, and took neither food nor drink." Ac 9:9

3. One to a Three Day Fasting Schedule

There are many different ways to set up a fasting schedule but some people like a structured one to follow. As you get more experienced in fasting you can create your own schedule of liquid intake that works best for you. Water can be taken at anytime during a fast, usually the more the better.

OPTION ONE   - Drink water as Needed
    Day One and Day Two of the Fast

Breakfast, 7:00 - 8:00		- Fruit Juice (1-2 cups)
		- Water as needed
	10:00 - 11:00	- Juice (½ to 1 cup)
		- Water as needed
Lunch	12:00 - 1:00	- Vegetable Juice (1-2 cups)
		- Water as needed
	2:00 - 3:00	- Juice (½ to 1 cup)
		- Water as needed
Dinner	5:00 - 6:00	- Juice (1-2 cups)
		- Water as needed
	8:00 - 9:00	- Juice, 1 cup
		- Water as needed
Bedtime	10:00 - 11:00	- Water or Juice (½ to 1 cup)

Day Three of a three day fast for Option I

Breakfast, 7:00 - 8:00		- Fruit Juice (1-2 cups)
		- Water as needed
	10:00 - 11:00	- Water or Juice (½ to 1 cup)
		- Water as needed
Lunch	12:00 - 1:00	- Vegetable Juice (1-2 cups)
		- Water as needed
		- A piece of fruit such as an apple, orange or stewed tomatoes.
		- Water as needed
	2:00 - 3:00	- Juice, 1 cup
		- A piece of fruit such as an apple, orange or

41

		stewed tomatoes.
		- Water as needed
Dinner	6:00 - 7:00	- Juice (1-2 cups)
		- A small salad or soup
		- Water as needed
	8:00 - 9:00	- Juice, 1 cup
		- Water as needed
Bedtime	10:00 - 11:00	- Water or Juice (½ to 1 cup)

OPTION TWO   for a FAST
Day One and Day Two of the Fast for Option Two

Take water as is needed on this option two.

Waking Up		- Glass of Fruit Juice
Breakfast,	7:00 - 8:00	- Two glasses of fruit juice
	8:00 - 9:00	- Water (½ to 1 cup)
	9:00 - 10:00	- Water or Juice (½ to 1 cup)
	10:00 - 11:00	- Water or Juice (½ to 1 cup)
	11:00 - 12:00	- Water or Juice (½ to 1 cup)
Lunch	12:00 - 1:00	- Vegetable Juice (1-2 cups)
	1:00 - 2:00	- Water or Juice (½ to 1 cup)
	2:00 - 3:00	- Juice, 1 cup
	3:00 - 4:00	- Water or Juice (½ to 1 cup)
	4:00 - 5:00	- Water or Juice (½ to 1 cup)
Dinner	5:00 - 6:00	- Juice (1-2 cups)
	6:00 - 7:00	- Water (½ to 1 cup)
	7:00 - 8:00	- Water or Juice (½ to 1 cup)
	8:00 - 9:00	- Juice, 1 cup
	9:00 - 10:00	- Water or Juice (½ to 1 cup)
Bedtime	10:00 - 11:00	- Water or Juice (½ to 1 cup)

Day Three of a three day fast for Option II

Waking Up		- Glass of Fruit Juice
Breakfast,	7:00 - 8:00	- Two glasses of fruit juice
	8:00 - 9:00	- Water (½ to 1 cup)
	9:00 - 10:00	- Water or Juice (½ to 1 cup)
	10:00 - 11:00	- Water or Juice (½ to 1 cup)

42

Lunch	11:00 - 12:00	-	Vegetable Juice (1-2 cups)
		-	A piece of fruit such as: apple, orange or stewed tomatoes.
	12:00 - 1:00	-	Water (½ to 1 cup)
	1:00 - 2:00	-	Water or Juice (½ to 1 cup)
	2:00 - 3:00	-	Juice, 1 cup
	3:00 - 4:00	-	Water or Juice (½ to 1 cup)
		-	A piece of fruit such as: apple, orange or stewed tomatoes.
	4:00 - 5:00	-	Water or Juice (½ to 1 cup)
Dinner	5:00 - 6:00	-	Juice (1-2 cups)
	6:00 - 7:00	-	Water (½ to 1 cup)
		-	A small salad or soup
	7:00 - 8:00	-	Water or Juice (½ to 1 cup)
	8:00 - 9:00	-	Juice, 1 cup
	9:00 - 10:00	-	Water or Juice (½ to 1 cup)
Bedtime	10:00 - 11:00	-	Water or Juice (½ to 1 cup)

OPTION III - Create Your Own Fast.

Option III takes Option I or II as a reference point and you create your own fasting schedule. Read and reread the teachings in this book to become aware of the basic principles of fasting and keep them in mind when you are creating your own fasting schedule. Fasting is a discipline and when you are able to follow your heart, listen to your body then try option III.

I have to admit that I have never used a fasting schedule since I always developed the fast and drank the juices, as my body needed them. Even though I am disciplined and try to drink something once or twice and hour, I usually do it according to what I feel I need rather than to follow a schedule. But some people need a schedule especially in the beginning when learning to fast. Thus learn to follow your heart and in this case your stomach and use these schedules as a guide to a fasting schedule, then listen inwardly.

4. Seven to Ten Day Fasting Schedule

Either Option One or Option Two or Option Three can be used for the seven to ten day fast but additional things are needed after the second day for a longer fast.

This is merely an outline and the next section goes into detail about a seven day fast schedule. Study the following section before coming back to this schedule and then adapt as is needed. Different people will have slightly different schedules.

Day one and day two have been gone over in detail. Thus here we are starting with day three.

Third Day of a Long Fast to empty the bowels.
Waking Up - Two Glasses of Prune Juice
Breakfast, 7:00 - 8:00 - Two Glasses of Prune Juice
Option I, II or III for your schedule.

Fourth Day of a Long Fast.
Option I, II or III for your schedule.
Broths and/or Green Drink
and/or Carrot Juice

Fifth Day of a Long Fast.
Option I, II or III for your schedule.
Broths and/or Green Drink
and/or Carrot Juice

Sixth Day of a Long Fast.
Option I, II or III for your schedule.
Broths and/or Green Drink
and/or Carrot Juice

Seventh Day of a Long Fast.
>   Option I, II or III for your schedule.
>   Broths and/or Green Drink
>   and/or Carrot Juice

Eighth to Tenth Day - if taken this long
>   Same as Seventh Day

First Day of Breaking a Long Fast.
>   Option I, II or III for your schedule.
>   Stewed Tomatoes, an Orange or Apple

Second Day of Breaking a Long Fast.
>   Option I, II or III for your schedule.
>   Stewed Tomatoes, an Orange or Apple
>   Small amounts of food once or twice.

Third Day of Breaking a Long Fast.
>   Option I, II or III as is needed.
>   Small amounts of food two or three times.

IV. The Seven to Ten Day Juice Fast

At the death of Saul, "they fasted for seven days."
1 Ch 10:12, 1 Sam 31:13

1. The Juice Fasting Programs

A seven day juice fasting program is spoken of in this book but oftentimes the terminology of 7 to 10 day fasting program will be used. Coming off a seven day fast may last for one or two or three more days, making it an 8, 9 or 10 day fast. Then a seven day fast will take three days to come off of it, as would an eight or nine or ten day fast.

Dr. Airola and Dr. Bragg both emphasize 7 to 10 day fasts, where as Dr. Walker only emphasizes a 6 to 7 day fast before breaking it. Most people who read this book are just learning to fast and have little experience in long fast. Seven days on a fast is enough for the average person. After gaining some experience for several seven day fasts, you can try for a few days more if your body and your spirit encourage you too. A seven day fast is sufficient for most people, longer 8-10 day fasts can be helpful and therapeutic, if they are done right. For fasts longer than 10 days a person should either be experienced or under guidance. After about twenty years of experience in 7 to 10 day fasts, I have found a 7 day fast is sufficient most of the time, but sometimes I do 8 or 9 days.

Thus for a seven day fast, fast for seven days and break the fast on the eight day. The eighth, ninth and tenth days are transitional days going back to normal eating. The eight day is still a fast day only with a little vegetables and fruit. But if needed you could start breaking the fast on the seventh day and still call it a seven day fast. Do what you are comfortable with.

In Dr. Paavo Airola's outlined in his book, his
program[49] for juice fasting:
1. Upon rising an enema,
2. Dry brush massage followed by a hot-cold
   Shower,
3. At 9:00 a cup of herb tea - warm not hot. He
   suggests,   peppermint, chamomile, or rose hips.
4. At 11:00 a glass of freshly-pressed fruit juice,
   diluted fifty-fifty with water.
5. Walk or mild exercise, spa or massage or
   sunbathing.
6. At 1:00 a glass of freshly made vegetable juice or
   a cup of vegetable broth.
7. At 1:30 to 4:00 rest in bed.
8. At 4:00 a Cup of herb tea.
9. Walk, therapeutic baths, light exercise or other
   treatments.
10. At 7:00 a glass of diluted vegetable or fruit juices, or
    a cup of vegetable broth.

He advises to drink plain lukewarm water or mineral
water if thirsty (two to three glasses total). The total liquid
intake should be 6 to 8 glasses and if thirsty then drink more.

Jim recommends the juice fast for long fasts and
either a juice fast or a water fast for one to three day fasts. I
do not recommend any specific daily regime to juice fasting
but have suggestions on what works best. I do recommend a
weekly regime on a 7-10 day fast since certain nutrients and
activities are helpful in not necessary.

Over the course of a week I recommend that it is best to
have a combination of;
   1. Both fruit and vegetable juices, a lot, daily.
   2. Juice made with a juicer at least once a day.
   3. Broths at least two or three times, for potassium
      and minerals.

4. Green juices or greens added to the broth for chlorophyll at least twice (celery, cucumber or leafy vegetable). Carrot juice recommended.
5. Enema's once or twice (more if needed).
6. Sunshine and fresh air, prayer time and relaxation.
7. Go to work at your job as you normally would.

Drinking water every day is also a must. Diluting the juices with water is highly recommended during a fast. Juices are very concentrated fruit sugar and drinking water and not only juice is needed during a fast.

For a juice fast, I recommend a steady diet of juices on a juice fast. Drink as much juice and water as you feel the need to. Usually first thing in the morning is a great time to do some juicing and make fresh apple juice or cantaloupe juice or other fruit juice. Then once or twice an hour have another glass of juice, if thirsty. Sometime in the late morning, around lunch time or in the afternoon have some tomato or V-8 juice or other vegetable juice, then go back to fruit juicing. Store bought bottled juice is good to use but at least once a day (morning and/or evening) use a juice machine to make some fresh juice. Then use a broth, perhaps in the evening, several times a week.

2. The Juice Fast

It is best not to mix fruit and vegetable juices since they are made up of different enzymes which could fight with each other in the stomach. Fruits and vegetables require different enzyme combinations for their effective digestion. If you drink fruit juices in the morning, then switch for an hour or more drink vegetable juices and then go back to fruit juices. However you drink your juices, drink the fruit juices at a separate time from the vegetable juices. Drink a variety of different juices and try to listen inwardly as to which ones your body desires, not your fleshy desires. What is your heart within you suggesting that you drink.

The different types of juices could include; orange juice, tomato juice, apple juice, prune juice and other standards that you could buy in the grocery store. But going to the health food store will give a larger variety such as: Mountain Apricot Juice; Banana Casablanca, Very Veggie (vegetable cocktail), Mega C (strawberry and juices), Pomegranate, Watermelon, Raspberry Cherry, Cape Cod Cranberry, Cranberry, Cranberry Lemonade, Organic Prune, Concord Grape, Mountain Raspberry, Organic Vegetable, Organic Orange-Pineapple-Banana, Papaya Nectar, Rio Red Grapefruit, Cranberry Orange, Blueberry Lemonade. Boysenberry Nectar, Oregon Berry, 24 Carrot Orange. And then sometimes you can mix the juices to come up with a completely different flavor.

There are many good juices that can be juiced in a mixer such as apple or carrot. Some of the vegetable juices are easier to drink if mixed together: such as celery-cucumber-squash juice. A great breakfast juice could be apple juice, cantaloupe juice, or honeydew Mellon juice.

When juicing, add a little water to the juicer when making the juice, especially at the end of the juicing session to get all the juice out of the juicer. When juicing it is best to drink freshly made juice but after you have had a glass or two save yourself some time and make an extra glass or two and keep it in the refrigerator. But fresh juice should be drunk within several hours and not left overnight or for more than 24 hours or it will start to breakdown and lose its nutritional value.

It is best to dilute the juices. Most juices are very concentrated and that amount of fruit sugar could be difficult on your system. Thus diluting the juice with water is beneficial. In a glass add 50% juice and 50% water or 75% juice and 25% water or whatever you feel comfortable with. It is also easier on the pocketbook since juice fasting, especially if you buy health food store juices, can be expensive and by doing a 50/50 it doubles the amount of juice to drink. And it is necessary to drink some water throughout the day and not just concentrated juices.

Keep several different kinds of juices in your refrigerator. That way you will be able to choose the one you feel drawn to, when you go to have a glass of juice. And have one or two different herbal teas available in case you want to have a cup of herb tea. A cup of herb tea with honey can be a nice change from drinking juices and broths all day long.

Let me (Jim) make it perfectly clear that all these different juices are not needed to go on a long fast. I know of one woman who went on a long fast of 14 days just on apple juice. Using all these different juices is the way I like to do juice fasting because it is fun to drink all the different kinds of juices; and also because the variety can give a wide range of nutrient, vitamins and minerals, which replenishes the body. Fasting helps to get rid of the toxins and poisons in the system while juices replenishes the body's cellular needs.

Does this mean that juice fasting is better than water fasting? Yes and No, that's a big debate and there are good points on both sides. While juice fasting gives nutrients to the body, those in water fasting would say that these nutrients are replaced as soon as you start eating. The real question is which one is the Lord calling you to do? Follow your heart and see.

Some people may have problems juice fasting because they have blood sugar problems (hypo- or hyper-glycemic, etc.) and may not be able to fast at all. In these cases they should try diluting the juices 25% juice to 75% water or 10% juice to 90% water. If nothing else the juice will give the water some taste so that you desire and enjoy drinking more fluids. Whether it is water or juice, drinking fluids is needed to help flush out your system and cleanse you of toxins.

Drinks that should be avoided include; coffee contains caffeine and tea contains tannic acid which is stimulants. Milk and milk products contain protein. The non-caloric soft drinks are artificially sweetened and contain chemicals. Any kind of soft drink or alcohol drink should also be avoided. These drinks excite the nervous system, start acid secretions in the stomach and stir up hunger. And they do not help the process of purification and elimination.

Most major grocery store buy juices are pasteurized and thus cooked over a 130 degrees. This high temperature kills the enzymes and just about anything else organic in these juices. Besides a lot of these juices is really not fruit juice. Buying juice in the health food stores is the best option, yet many of these are pasteurized too, but hopefully, flash pasteurized and not as high a temperature.

The healthier a person becomes by getting rid of the toxins and poisons in his body the more he can dilute the juice with water. Eventually he would be down to 95% water and 5% juice and he might as well switch over to just water fasting. The science of Juice fasting started this century and is a cultural remedy for our sick society and its dietary habits. The water fast could be considered a superior fast over juice fasting for a perfectly healthy person who has no toxins or poisons in their body. But most people cannot make that claim and thus juice fasting helps us in our weakness and problematic physiological conditions.

3. Vegetable broths

Dr. Airola emphasizes vegetable broths along with juices. "Vegetable broth is one of the standard beverages during fasting in all biological clinics in Europe. Fasting patients at our Spa receive a large glass of vegetable broth first thing in the morning and before going to bed. It is a cleansing and alkalizing drink which supplies a great amount of vitamins and particularly minerals, which are so important for establishing and normalizing a proper chemical balance in the tissues during fasting. Vegetable broth is particularly rich in the mineral potassium."[50]

He recommends that the broth be made up of: 2 large potatoes, 1 cup of carrots, 1 cup of red beets, 1 cup of celery and 1 cup of any other vegetable: turnips, parsley, cabbage, beet tops, turnip tops or a little of everything. All of these are chopped, sliced or shredded. Cover and cook slowly in one and one-half quarts of water. Cook for an hour, let stand for an hour; strain, cool until warm and serve. Refrigerate the leftovers and warm before serving.

Dr. Airola states that; "a satisfactory broth can be made with only potatoes, beets, carrots, and celery, consisting of approximately 50% potatoes, 20% carrots, 15% beets and 15% celery."[51]

I recommend vegetable broths as a necessary part of a 7 to 10 day juice fast. They are a little bit of work but they really taste good after drinking juices all day. A lot of juices are very acidic and a vegetable broth is very alkaline so it helps to balance out the blood chemistry. I cut all the vegetables up into small pieces, cook the broth for about 20 minutes, strain it and drink it while it is still hot. Try to get at least two full cups of broth so you need about a quart of water since some will be absorbed and some will boil away.

The way that I make the broths is often different then Dr. Airola's recommendation. Usually I juice carrots, cucumbers and celery during a fast so I seldom add them into a broth. Potato's, beets and greens are probably the essential vegetables. Here are five different broths that I made up for the 7-10 day or longer fasts I have been on, when I was writing this section of the book:
  1) 1 potato; 1 onion; 1 sweet potato; some parsley and
       some spinach.

2) 1 red potato; 1 onion; ½ sweet potato; ½ beet; 2
    carrots; 2 celery;
  some parsley and some spinach.
3) 2 red potatoes; 1 onion; ½ beet; 2 celery; some parsley
    and spinach.
4) 1 red potato; 1 sweet potato; 1/4 beet; several carrots;
    spinach
5) 1 red potato, 1 sweet potato, ½ celery stock, 1 red
    onion, 3 cloves garlic, 1 red pepper, 3 small
    tomatoes, 6 or so asparagus, 1 lemon, 1 lime, 1
    small yellow and also green squash, teaspoon of
    flax seed oil, little salt and dulse and kelp granules.

Two basic types of broths can be made a potato broth
and a cabbage broth; this can separate the vegetable starches.

6) A potato broth (one potato, some of the rest: yam,
    onion, garlic, orange pepper, beet).
7) A cabbage broth (cabbage, asparagus, broccoli, tomato,
    add kale or spinach).

Also adding to a warm drink or a broth frozen
wheatgrass cubes or a teaspoon of wheatgrass is good. So
experiment and make up your own vegetable broth.

4. Starting a Long Fast

Dr. Airola recommends preparing oneself for a fast
with a short 2 or 3 day cleansing diet when you eat raw fruits
and vegetables. Then start a fast with a bowel cleansing
purgative such as Glauber's salts or castor oil. On the first
day of the fast an hour or two before an enema, two
tablespoons of pure castor oil should be taken with water and
half a lemon added. Or he suggests beginning the fast
without a purgative and just using a double enema.

The fasting writer Steve Meyerowitz recommends a
pre-fast diet. "A typical pre-fast diet may consist of a day of

cooked vegetables, salads, fruits and juices on the first day. Any food in these categories is acceptable, but it is still a limited diet because it excludes grains, breads, and dairy, fish and flesh foods. Day two is usually slightly more limited with only raw salads, fruits and juices. Day three might just be limited to fruits and juices. Each day is progressively more restricted up to the day of the fast. The fruits and vegetables are of course, eaten separately, e.g., fruits for lunch, vegetables for dinner. If time is limited and you are a seasoned faster, you may choose a one day pre-fast, which might turn out to be a day of salads or a day of fruits and juices. Always keep the juices and water in your pre-fast diet since they are the major elements of the actual fast."[52]

Usually the day before a fast I start preparing for the fast by staying away from heavy foods and starches and junky food. And the evening before I eat a light meal. But at least a week or two before the long fast I start preparing myself psychologically. I note the week and day that I want to start the fast and start clearing my schedule and inwardly start looking forward to doing a long fast.

I recommend starting a fast by not eating a lot. Perhaps for some people eating a special diet to prepare for a fast and using a purgative and an enema to start a fast may be helpful. But the easiest way is to stop eating the night before and in the morning start drinking juices. Sometimes it is best not to eat a big meal the night before since it will make starting a fast difficult in the morning, but I have eaten a big meal then started a long fast and it was fine, so follow your heart. Eating light the day before with a lot of fruits and vegetables is a good recommendation.

The question could be asked, How can I fast and yet escape the feelings of hunger during the first three days? Dr. Bragg has a great answer for this question. "And I have only one answer 'Just Grin and Bear.' 'I tried a fast once, but I got so weak, and felt so miserable, I just had to start eating.' This is another statement I often hear. Nowhere in this book

(Bragg) have I stated that fasting is easy. Eating has become such an important part of people's lives that if you take food away from them, and start them on a fast, they experience many mental and physical reactions. That is the very reason why fasting is not popular."[53]

The first day or two or three of a fast is oftentimes the most difficult part of the fast because your body is still craving food. And thus you may have hunger pains for the first few days of the fast. Drinking a lot of juice can help overcome these hunger pains and discomfort. I can remember experiencing hunger pains the first few times I fasted but that seldom happens to me anymore, partly because I drink so much juice which covers up hunger. I think it is also partly a psycho-physiological reaction. So just grin and bear it.

Sometimes negative symptoms can occur on a long fast such as: bad breath, stuffy or running nose; farting; headache; lightness in the head; a rash; acne; weakness; nausea; diarrhea; muscle aches or cramps; etc. These can be caused by numerous reasons, especially which poisons and toxins are leaving the system. But they are usually fleeting.

It is helpful to plan a fast from one weekend to the next. If you start a fast on a Saturday then the first two days, which may be difficult, are on the weekend. A seven day fast would end on the following Friday when you can break it sometime during the day or that evening. Then the weekend again is the time of breaking the fast and starting to eat again, which can be a difficult part of the fast.

Prune Juice should be used on the second or third day of a long fast. On the second day of a fast I usually drink a quart of prune juice in the morning. Drink two glasses and an hour or so later drink two more glasses. This will help to flush out your bowels.

It might be a wise caution to bring an extra pair of underwear to work or wear two pairs (or do both) after drinking prune juice. A long fast may cause some farting and after you drink prune juice a little liquid may come out when you fart. So for a couple of hours after drinking the prune juice, be aware. Diarrhea or loose stools may also occur the first couple of days.

It is best to dress warm during a fast or wear layers so you can peel some of them off. If you feel a little chilly that is normal since the body is used to eating not fasting.

Timing is important when doing a long fast, try to plan ahead and set aside a week that you're not busy and clear your schedule of activities. Once I wanted to do a fast at the end of the summer but things were too busy that summer, so I decided to wait till September but then September was too busy. Before I knew it I was into the middle of October before I just decided to start the fast, busy or not. I have done long fast when I was extremely busy and when it was more of a retreat, both work but the best thing to do is to try and set aside a week to ten days of retreat time. A fast works best if it is a retreat, a time set apart for you and the Lord.

5. Breaking a Long Fast

Both Dr. Paavo Airola and Dr. Paul Bragg advise that to fast longer than seven to ten days should be done under expert supervision.[54] I would agree that under ten days you could do a fast by yourself but over ten days you should either by under supervision or be experienced at fasting. Fasting for seven days and then breaking it is a good and easy time table to work with.

You want to come off the fast so slowly that this transition back to food is easy and uneventful, so that it just happens naturally. *Coming off the fast is the most difficult part of the fast and to come off it slowly is important.* Instead of waiting for the hunger to start, which usually happens during or after the seventh day, break the fast on the seventh or morning of the eight day. Then by a slow transition the hunger will occur naturally as you are engaged in the process of starting to eat again.

The day you break the fast is really still a fasting day since you'll be drinking juice all day and just eating a little fruit and vegetables. Thus if you feel anxious about it or start to feel hungry then go ahead and break the fast on the seventh day by starting the process on the seventh rather than on the eight day. *Having a goal of seven days also makes things easier since we are conditioned in our culture to reach a goal, it make us feel good when we can do that in fasting.*

Fasting until the hunger starts is the method that most fasting professionals use. But breaking the fast on a definite day, like the sixth or seventh or eighth day, hopefully a day or two before the hunger starts is just as efficient when the transition back to food is slow and natural. Thus sometime during the seventh day or morning of the eight you can break the fast, either early in the morning or later in the evening. Wait and see how you feel, physiologically and psychologically on the seventh or eighth day.

Thus you might want to break the fast on the sixth day if you feel hunger or just feel you want to break it then, but try to wait until the morning of the seventh day. Then if you're feeling great, the morning of the 7th day, continue on the juice fast throughout the 7th day and break it in the evening or the next morning. If you want to wait until the morning of the eight day before breaking it then do that. Learn to listen to your body and then follow your heart.

Knowing the need to break a fast comes from both the body and soul (mind, emotions and will). Physiologically you may experience hunger, a desire for food or protein, juice is not enough anymore, your craving after thicker heavier juices. Emotionally there may be mood swings, feeling down or afraid, a lot of will power to continue the fast, negative emotions such as sadness or depression. When one or more of these symptoms starts to occur throughout the day (physiological or psychological) then it could be time to break the fast.

How a person breaks a fast is very important. It takes more disciple to break a fast then to start it. And if the fast is broken improperly it can be painful and disruptive to your system. There are different ways to break the long fast but the main rule is to only eat a little at a time, then wait before eating more. Breaking a fast involves "Will Power".

The following will relate what the various fasting experts say about fasting. **All of these doctors cited below break the fast with tomato's, apples and oranges.** And three of them: Dr. Bragg, Dr. Shelton and Dr. Hazzard recommend using a tomato to break the fast.

Dr. Airola writes on breaking a long fast. "Whether you're fast will turn out to be a success or a failure will depend largely on how you break your fast. Breaking a fast is the most significant phase of it. The beneficial effect of fasting could be totally undone if the fast is broken incorrectly! As Dr. Otto H. F. Buchinger says: 'Even a fool can fast, but only a wise man knows how to break the fast properly and to build up properly after the fast!'"

Dr. Airola continues: "The main rules from breaking a fast are: 1. Do not overeat! 2. Eat slowly and chew your food extremely well. 3. Take several days of gradual transition to the normal diet. First day: Eat one whole apple in the morning and a very small bowl or raw vegetable salad at lunch, in addition to the usual juice and broth menu. Second day: Soaked prunes or figs (with the soaking water) for breakfast; Small bowl of fresh vegetable salad for lunch; Vegetable soup made without salt at dinner; Two apples eaten between meals. All this is in addition to the usual

juices and broths. Third day: As second day, but add a glass
of yogurt and a few raw nuts for breakfast. Increase the salad
portion at lunch, and add a boiled or baked potato. A slice of
whole grain bread with butter and a slice of cheese with soup
at evening. "[55]   On the fourth day he states that you can start
eating normally and should start a build-up diet of natural
foods.

Dr. Airola's has three points on breaking a fast, they
are a must: If you do not eat slowly and chew your food up
or if you eat too much then you will suffer. Your intestinal
track has shrunk and needs to open up slowly. Dr. Airola
concludes saying, "But first and foremost, keep always in
mind the first rule of breaking the fast: do not overeat! This
rule also happens to be the first rule of keeping healthy and
staying younger longer."[56]

Dr. Bragg recommends breaking a fast this way.
"Around 5 o'clock of the 7th day of the fast, peel 4 or 5
medium sized tomatoes, cut them up, bring them to a boil and
then turn off the heat, and when they are cool enough to eat,
have as many as you desire."[57] The next morning he
recommends a salad of grated carrots and grated cabbage,
with half an orange squeezed over it, then some steamed
greens and peeled tomatoes and some toast thoroughly dry.

Dr. Otto H.F. Buchinger, M.D. writes on breaking a
fast. "From many years' experience the fresh apple has
definitely proved the best way of introducing the breaking of
the fast. Its organic trace materials are conveyed to the
organism in the natural and unrepeated form in which pectin
and the core have a function promoting peristaltic
movement."[58] He states to break the fast in the morning
with an apple, then have another apple in the afternoon. And
in the evening have a little plain potato soup.

Dr. Allan Cott, M.D., believes in water fasts with
water only. He suggests breaking a fast, of two days or
longer, the first day after the fast; "In the morning mix two

quarts of water with one quart of orange juice or apricot juice. Sip two teaspoonfuls of the mixture every five or ten minutes in the first hour after breaking the fast. Sip teaspoonfuls at regular intervals throughout the day, but make sure the concoction lasts until bedtime."[59] The second day he recommends using undiluted juice. Breaking a fast with juice is a common approach.

Dr. Herbert Shelton states, "that fasts may be broken on whatever food is available, providing sufficient caution is observed." "Almost every advocate of fasting has evolved his own techniques for breaking a fast. There seems to be a tendency for each man to assume that his own techniques are best. There may be several techniques, each one of which is as good as the others. The chief requirement in breaking a fast is to use simple, wholesome food and feed this in keeping with the limited digestive capacity of the faster. Time is required for the digestive secretions to begin to be produced in normal amounts and, until they are secreted in normal quantities, the ability to digest food is limited."[60]

Some people encourage breaking a fast with juices and others breaking a fast with foods. Dr. Shelton writes of an associate Dr. Virginia Vetrano who thoroughly tested both methods of breaking a fast and found that breaking a fast with food was superior to breaking a fast with juices. "For breaking a long fast, she served one-half orange every two hours, the first day. The second day, have a whole orange every two hours. The second day may be varied in the following manner. At 8 a.m. one may have one orange; at 10 a.m., one apple; at 12:00 noon, one pear; at 2p.m., one tomato; at 4p.m., one-half grapefruit; and at 6 p.m. one orange. It is best the first day after a long fast to stay with one type of fruit. The second day, if all goes well, every two hours the faster may have a different fruit in season, providing it is as small as one orange."[61] The suggestion of using a whole orange or whole tomato with a maximum of six a day is also suggested.

Dr. Linda Hazzard, D.O. writes on breaking a fast. "In the ordinary instance a successfully completed fast should be broken by the ingestion of the juices of ripe fruit or of broths prepared from vegetables. The juices of fruits that are fully ripened are most easily changed in mouth and stomach for subsequent digestive processes, and there is but small effort in handling them. The same reasoning is applicable to the use of vegetable broths, strained through a coarse kitchen sieve so as to remove fibrous material and hard solid particles. There are many vegetables that lend themselves readily to the preparation of these broths, and, when the latter are made as indicated so as to exclude all but finely comminuted solid matter, they are easily digested and their products are assimilated promptly and without difficulty. When using the juices of fruit to break a fast, it is suggested that those of sweet fruit be not mixed with those of acid. One fruit as a time is the rule. At first the broths should be confined in preparation to one vegetable, such as the tomato or the onion. Later they may be varied in ingredients, and combinations may be made of two or three kinds. The tomato is perhaps the one vegetable that lends itself most satisfactorily to the breaking of a fast, and it is in the constant use for this purpose by the author."[62]

As stated above, all of these doctors just cited break the fast with tomato's, apples and oranges. And three of them: Dr. Bragg, Dr. Shelton and Dr. Hazzard recommend using a tomato to break the fast.

I have tried many different ways of breaking a long fast and have found that boiling several tomatoes (like Dr. Bragg suggests) and eating them is the best way. The reason this works (stewed tomatoes) is because the alkaline content of the tomatoes helps to open up the intestinal tract.

Starting a fast becomes easy and automatic after a few years of fasting. But coming off of a fast takes discipline and patience to do it right even after twenty years of fasting.

A basic schedule could be:

1. Once you have decided to break a fast then cook one or two tomato's for 5 to 10 minutes, until they are soft. Or you could just eat them raw and uncooked. Slowly eat the tomatos.
2. Have some juice.
3. Wait until lunch and have one or two more stewed tomatoes or raw tomatos.
4. Have some juice in between.
5. At dinner have some more uncooked or stewed tomatoes and peel a half an apple or orange and slowly eat the apple, chew it up very well before swallowing it.
6. Have some juice in between.
7. The next morning have a piece of fruit and a stewed tomato.
8. Have some juice in between.
9. At lunch have a small bowl of fruit salad or broth-soup.
10. Continue to slowly add food the next day.

A program like this should be spread out over a whole day. The purpose is to slowly open up your intestines. The second day starches and carbohydrates could be introduced but it is really better to wait till the third day.

The broth-soup could be made up of numerous different ingredients mostly it should be of the vegetables that you were using to make broths all week long with. The one that I made up during this writing was;

5 cups water, 2 red potatoes, 1 beet, 3 scallions, ½ onion, 3 small carrots, parsley, cabbage, ½ teaspoon of sea salt. (or create your own)

Cook it 20 minutes or until the potatoes, carrots and cabbage are soft.

One reason this longer fast is referred to as a 7 to 10 day fast is because it usually takes about three days to come off the fast and start eating normally. The day that you break the fast is really like a fast day. Such as if you break the fast at lunch time with stewed tomatoes you will still drink juice the rest of the afternoon and evening and have a little salad or something in the evening. This is like a fast day and should probably be referred to as one.

Here is a good example of how to break a seven day fast. It is different from the one described above but it is basically the same. The key is to have fruits and vegetables for the first two days of coming off the fast.

Break the fast with two stewed tomatoes or;

Morning 8th day   - one stewed tomato &
                                a third of an apple.

Lunch 8th day   - 2 stewed tomatoes &
                                a third of an apple.

Snack 8th day   - a third of an apple.

Dinner 8th day   - 2 stewed tomatos
                                little lettuce

Morning 9th day   - 2 stewed tomatos
                                A quarter of cantaloupe

Lunch 9th day   - 1 stewed tomato
                                2 pieces lettuce
                                a third cucumber

Snack   - a pear

Dinner 9th day   - 1 stewed tomato
                                2 pieces lettuce
                                little parsley
                                little broccoli

Morning 10th day   - a quarter cantaloupe
                                a little bowl of oatmeal

Snack 10th day - apple

Lunch 10th day   - 2 pieces lettuce
                                little parsley
                                little broccoli
                                little bread with peanut butter

The key is that the day you break the fast is really still a fast day just with a little fruit and vegetables. The second day of breaking the fast is still juice and a little more fruit and vegetables. Not until the third day should carbohydrates and proteins are introduced. And then only in small amounts should non fruits and vegetables be introduced.

It takes at least three days to come off a seven day fast. The transition back to eating is really a very important part of the fast and takes the most patience and discipline, so that you do not binge and pig out.

6. Your Personal Fasting Program

I agree with the benefits of a 7 to 10 day fast at least once or twice a year. Here's a summary of four of the fasting orientations mentioned in this book.

Paul Bragg recommends that a 7 to 10 day fast
be taken four times a year.
Paavo Airola recommends that a 7 to 10 day fast
be taken once or twice a year.
Norman Walker recommends a 6 to 7 day fast.
James Tibbetts recommends a 7-10 day fast
be taken two or three or four times a year
or do longer 14-21 day fast in place of
two 7 day fast.

In addition to a weekly one day fast (which could be a juice or fruit or smoothie fast) and two or three 7- 10 day fasts I would recommend doing a longer 14 to 21 day fast once a year in place of the 7 day fast. This would give three to four times of fasting a year. This gives a spring, summer, fall and winter time of fasting.

Start off doing one day a week cleanses, then trying a 7- 10 day fast. After you get comfortable with the 7 day juice fast move onto trying a 14 to 21 day juice fast.

A lot of fasting experts tend to emphasis a 7 to 10 day fast. But a 7 day fast is usually sufficient and then it usually takes 3 days to come off a fast which ends up being a ten day fasting period. Sometimes it is helpful to set a goal to do a 7 day fast and fit that into your schedule. But if you're inspired to go beyond 7 days to 8 or 9 or 10 days follow the Spirit's lead; doing the extra day or two on a fast can be very helpful.

People with expertise in fasting recommend doing a weekly one day fast and a yearly seven day fast, though how many times a year a person should do a seven day fast differs among the experts, I recommend at least two a year.

Paul Bragg makes an interesting comment that he has led people on fast for over forty years and came to the conclusion that the long three and four week fasts were good but doing four seven day fasts a year was better. Thus after a life time of experience of fasting he came to the conclusion that several shorter 7 to 10 day fasts were better than one long 21 to 28 day fast every year.

"Jehoshaphat was alarmed and resolved to have recourse to Yahweh; he proclaimed a fast for all Judah."
2 Ch 20:3

V. Questions and Answers on Fasting

"Prayer with fasting and alms with right conduct are better than riches with iniquity." Tb 12:8

1.   Question - Should I own a juicer?
      Answer -Yes, to do a long fast a juicer is helpful for juicing. You can buy the bottled juices that are out there but you will miss the benefit and delight of fresh made juices. There are a lot of bottled fruit juice drinks but it is hard to get good vegetable juice drinks that are fresh. Always peel and wash the fruits and vegetables before juicing them. But if you do not have or cannot afford a juicer just use bottled juice.

2.   Question - Should I buy supermarket juices or health food store juices?
      Answer - Health food store juices are usually organic and contain more real juice in them. Supermarket juices are usually refined and highly purified for a longer shelf life and usually contain a lot of sweeteners. There is a noticeable difference between supermarket juices and health food store juices. Health food store bought juices are the better choice. The health food store juices are usually very concentrated (and expensive) so dilute them with water, as your taste prefers.

3.   Question - Should I go to work on a 7 to 10 day fast?
      Answer - Sure, why not. Hard physical labor or exercise would be difficult to do but most jobs can easily accommodate a 7 day fast.

4.   Question - What type of work is best to do on a fast?
      Answer - Any kind of work is O.K. but reading, writing, thinking type of work is the easiest to do. A clarity

of thought and imagination are usually found in a fast. In fact, as I type this Question and Answer I am on the 6th day of a juice fast.

The fasting program that I recommend in this book is designed around working a regular eight hour a day job. That is why I recommend juicing in the morning and evening and drinking bottled juice in between. Juice gives fruit sugar that goes directly into the bloodstream and gives energy to do a normal day's workload.

5.   Question - How long and how many times should one fast?
     Answer   - This question has been partly answered above in this book. But fasting is an individual thing and needs to be decided upon by each individual. At least once or twice a year go on a 7 to 10 day fast, and once a week for a 24-36 hour fast is often best.

6.   Question - Can Fasting lengthen one's life span?
     Answer   - A prolonged life span through fasting and diet is a statement made by all the major promoters fasting and health diets. Studies have shown that rats fed on a low protein diet one day and then fasted the next lived 50% longer then normally fed rats. A major study on the Seventh Day Adventists in California showed that they lived an average of ten years longer than the average Californian.

7.   Question - Will my thinking be O.K. during a fast?
     Answer   - You may have a sense of clarity of thought and a heighten awareness by the fast. Eating foods can bring a heaviness whereas fasting might bring a sense of lightness. Also your sense of smell and taste might be heighten.

8.   Question - Since I have not eaten for a week, do I have to eat double after a fast, to make up for lost time?
     Answer   - No, hunger is not cumulative and after a fast you are not trying to make up for lost time.

9.   Question - Can Fasting help overweight problems?
        Answer   - Yes, there are many doctors and nearly all
health clinics help people to reduce weight through fasting.
Perhaps the best way to get started to develop your own,
Personal Fasting Program, as outlined in this book and try it
for several months to a year.

10.   Question - Can Fasting help underweight people?
        Answer   - Ironically, Yes, since fasting helps cleans
the whole gastrointestinal track increasing its ability to
absorb food and nutrients. A 7-10 day juice fast is good for
underweight people but short fasts can be very helpful, too.
Both Dr. Bragg and Dr. Airola state that fasting can help
underweight people.

11.   Question - What is the very best program for fasting?
        Answer   - The very best program for fasting is your
own Personal Fasting Program practiced with faith and
sincerity. Everyone is unique and has different biochemistry
and problems. There is no fasting program that is the ideal
fasting program. Find out what works best for you, that is
what God is calling you to do.

12.   Question - Can fasting give muscle cramps?
        Answer   - Yes, muscle cramps can occur but that
possibly means that you are releasing a lot of toxins and
poisons or perhaps you do not have enough salt or potassium,
thus the need for broths. Some bottled vegetable juices like
tomato juice or V-8 has salt in it. Health food juices would
have sea salt which is better than regular salt.

13.   Question - Can a person have sex during a fast?
        Answer   - Sure, why not, as long as it is with your
spouse and in moderation. Any kind of excessive exercise
should be avoided during a fast.

14.   Question - Does a person need to have a Personal
Fasting Program?

Answer   - Yes, if you ever want to make it into a lifestyle. Otherwise it will become something that you do now and then. And eventually you will fall away from the practice since you will come up with many reasons not to fast.

Spiritual reasons are not enough for a Personal Fasting Program, there needs to be acceptance that it is beneficial to your body too. It needs to become a personal disciple for health reasons too.

15.   Question - Has anyone ever died on a fast?
       Answer   - Yes on long fasts over 28 days, but it is very rare. Arnold Ehert writes of a 60 year old man who fasted 28 days and then when he broke the fast he had to be operated on and died shortly afterwards. It was breaking the fast improperly that killed him, not the fast itself. And the man was not properly prepared to fast that long for his age. The few deaths on long fasts over 30 days are because of complications or illness.

That is why long fasts over three weeks should be done under professional supervision. A healthy person on a long fast over two to three weeks has little to nothing to worry about, it's those who are older and/or have serious illness that needs to be concerned. But a 7 to 10 day fast is safe, even a 14 to 21 day fast is safe, so do not worry about it, be happy and enjoy it!

16.   Question - On a long fast, how do I know if it is time
   to break a fast?
       Answer -   There are different indications such as: desire for food or a strong hunger; desire to have heavier thicker juice drinks; a desire for protein, prolonged weakness or nausea; stressful work schedule arises; a gut level feeling or intuition; the time is up for a long fast and your goal is reached (for example seven days).

17.   Question - How do I know if I should juice fast, water fast or bread and water fast?
       Answer - Try them all and see for yourself. Some people prefer water fasting and others prefer juice fasting. It is partly a physiological decision and you will gravitate towards one or the other. For a small minority, bread and water fasting or penitential fasting may be their personal disciple. But the average healthy person should try to go with a water or a juice fasting discipline.

18.   Question - Can I brush my teeth during a fast?
       Answer   - Yes, just don't swallow the toothpaste.

19.   Question - Should I have ice cubes or very hot drinks on a fast?
       Answer - No, the stomach is already contracted on a fast. Having a warm drink is O.K. but a hot drink or ice cubes may irritate the stomach.

20.   Question - Can I drink coffee or tea, beer or wine during a fast.
       Answer - No. Coffee and most regular teas have caffeine. Alcoholic drinks and caffeine, and also milk stimulates the stomach to secrete acids. Avoid these drinks during a fast.

21.   Question - What's the average amount I should drink during a fast?
       Answer - Try to drink one glass of liquid an hour, water or juice. Sometime you may need more other times you may desire less.

22.   Question - Can I drink milk during a fast?
       Answer   - No. I once met a girl who used to fast on milk, she ending up with an ulcer. Milk is a protein and starts the digestive acids secreting in your stomach.

23.   Question - Should pregnant woman fast?

Answer   - No, it will not hurt the woman but it might hurt the developing child in the womb. Fasting during pregnancy or lactation should be avoided, unless under expert fasting supervision.

24.   Question - Should young children fast?
        Answer   - No, it could cause problems. I have not read any fasting expert that recommends children fast. Except under expert fasting supervision for serious illnesses.

25.   Question - Should I use vitamin pills during a fast?
        Answer - No, they are not needed since the juices are supplying you with what you need. If you do take vitamins, then only take water soluble vitamins.

26.   Question - Should a person fast if on drugs?
        Answer   - It depends what kind of drug but in general no a person on a drug should not fast and should seek expert advice. Drugs like aspirin and Tylenol should also be avoided.

27.   Question - Should a person fast if they are afflicted with diabetes, tuberculosis, or certain other advanced and debilitating diseases?
        Answer   - Maybe, a lengthy fast is not recommended unless under expert supervision, but fasting might help.

28.   Question - Why don't Medical Doctors recommend fasting?
        Answer   - The last I heard there was only one medical school in the country that requires a course in nutrition and no medical schools teach or practice fasting. Also there is not a lot of good objective scientific research done on fasting to back up the many theories of how it works. Most medical doctors are not trained in the science of fasting but naturopathic doctors have training in nutrition and often times in fasting. Most cities nowadays have a naturopathic doctor or two who could give advice.

29.   Question - Is there a best type of diet after finishing a fast?

    Answer - There is a best way to break a fast but there are many types of diets that you can go on after a fast. Every health food book has its own version of the "best" diet. But I believe the "best" diet is the one the Lord wants you to be on. There are probably only about a third of the foods in the average supermarket that I think are worth eating. You will have to seek inwardly what the Spirit is calling you to eat and how the Spirit wants you to prepare it.

30.   Question - Does fasting or eating have anything to do with love?

    Answer - Through fasting and diet a person and appreciate and learn to love their body. Love of God is the highest form of love, love of neighbor is the next and then love of one's self, (and one's body) would come next. Learning to love one's body through fasting and diet involves two basic principles; first 'giving' our bodies what the body needs and secondly 'receiving' with love what situations and others may give out to us. Of course receiving also means knowing when to say 'no thank you' or 'I have had enough'.

    "If anybody should destroy the temple of God, God will destroy him, because the temple of God is sacred, and you are the temple." 1 Cor 3.17

    "Your body, you know, is the temple of the Holy Spirit, who is in you since you received him from God."
                1 Cor 6 19

VI. Therapeutic Fasting

"He (Jesus) fasted for forty days and forty nights, after which he was very hungry." Mt 4:2   Afterwards, "Jesus, returned in the power of the Spirit to Galilee." Lk 4:14

Therapeutic fasting involves fasting longer than 10 days, at least two to three weeks. In Europe the standard therapeutic fast is about 21 days while in America it is about 28 days. Oftentimes the fast goes longer than 28 days but 40 days is usually considered the maximum. A seven to ten day fast can be healing but it's just beginning the process. Usually it is best to be under medical supervision but about the only thing they will do is to tell you to break the fast when you've gone long enough. This book is about a 7 to 10 day fast and not about leading a person into a long therapeutic fast. But knowing something about therapeutic fasting is good.

As you will see therapeutic fasting can heal most kinds of degenerative diseases. It can also be an excellent complementary approach to modern medicine.

1. Fasting to Lose Weight

During a 7 to 10 day fast a person can usually lose between 5 to 10 pounds. But after the fast they may gain some or all of the weight back after eating for several weeks. Fasting can take off weight but it is the diet that maintains the weight. A very heavy person could lose 5 lbs. a day at first which is probably because they lost 2 gallons of water at 8 lbs./gal.

The 7 to 10 day fast found in this book may not be of much help in losing a lot of weight, longer fasts or several 7 day fasts are usually needed. Instead of longer fast over ten days it might be better to do a series of 7 day fasts. Fast for 7 days then go back to eating for a few weeks then do another 7 day fast. Doing this several times might be healthier and more productive then one real long fast.

Today medical doctors and researchers have studied prolonged fasting in-depth with modern scientific methods. In one professional journal prolonged fasting among obese patients is discussed. It was found that physiological problems can occur in fasts over forty days. "Metabolic changes that occur in fasting patients were studied with special reference to those metabolic disturbances that might adversely affect the health of the patient.

"Fasting is an effective method of treating obesity, and no serious metabolic disturbances were encountered when the fast lasted less than 40 days. However, in prolonged fasting (i.e. periods greater than 40 days) electrolyte disorders, protein deficiency, normochromic anemia and mal-absorption of vitamin B12 were encountered."[63]

"As in previous studies by Bloom(1), Drenick et al. (2) and Thomson et al. (3), we found fasting an effective treatment for obesity, and one of our patients who fasted for 14 weeks lost 84 lb. In some cases the weight loss produced a dramatic improvement in the well-being of the patient."[64]

Some examples of weight loss during a water fast by three patients are indicated by the number of days fasting and the weight loss. Patient DS, Day 1-208; 14-197; 22-192; 32-185; 35-183; 41-176. Patient GS, Day 1-204; 9-196; 23-192; 40-176; 45-171. Postfast GS, Day 59-174; 69-175; 79-176. Patient FG, Day 1-250; 3-237; 9-231; 15-227; 19-224; 27-219; 30-216; 35-213; 42-208; 47-206. Thus within the first two weeks the three patients lost; 11 lbs., 11 lbs. and 23 lbs. respectively.

All eight patients (21-42 years) in this study gained weight initially but then the weight gain remained steady and substantially below the pre-fasting level. Breaking the fast was several days on fruit and milk drinks only, before they were introduced to a high protein-low carbohydrate diet. The first two days were difficult for all the patients and then they experienced no negative symptoms until about the 40th day. Up to about 40 days the moral was high and then after 40 days nausea and other symptoms were frequent. The patients lost approximately 0.8 lbs. daily, the first week was the greatest weight loss.[65]

2. Therapeutic Water Fasting

"Yet, when they were sick, I put sackcloth on,
I humbled my soul with fasting." Ps 35:13

A therapeutic fast is a fast undertaken for the purpose of healing and should be done under a doctor's supervision. A therapeutic fast is usually between 10 days and 40 days. Dr. Airola states that for therapeutic fasts, "The most common length of fasts in European clinics is 14 to 21 days. It would not be advisable to undertake a do-it-yourself fasting program for longer than one week or ten days."[66]

Dr. Airola and others have numerous examples of physical healings that came through fasting. One of the greats in fasting is, Dr. Herbert Shelton. In his book; *Fasting for the Health of It* he presents 100 case studies from 11 different doctors and Hygienic practitioners, that have been cured through fasting. Most of these cases are serious medical cases which were healed either partially or totally.[67]

a. Dr. Herbert Shelton

Of the 100 Case studies noted in Dr. Shelton's book: *Fasting for the Health of It*, some of the conditions that were cured or improved were as follows, the days fasted for that individual case are indicated. In some of the categories there were more than one patient who had that disease and fasted but each is only mentioned once.

Some of the conditions that were cured or improved were as follows, the days fasted for that individual case are indicated. This is taken from Dr. Shelton's book: *Fasting for the Health of It* [68]

Parkinson's disease (30, 14, 14 days)	insomnia (21 days),
multiple sclerosis (14 days),	bursitis (21 days),
colitis (10, 21, 10 days),	abdominal tumor (7 days),
depression (18 days),	alcoholism (26 days),
hypoglycemia (days),	gonorrhea (12 days),
high blood pressure (10 days),	brain tumor (8 days),
	headaches (22 days),
arthritis (10, 14, 10 days),	back pain (7, 8, 7 days),
diverticulitis (14, 21 days),	eczema (28, 10, 10 days),
obesity (10 days),	hemorrhoids (14 days),
drug addiction (10 days),	intestinal disorder (21 days),
high cholesterol (10 days),	angina (28 days),
kidney stones (10, 14 days),	cerebral stroke (25 days),
acne (10 days),	glaucoma (21 days),
Crohn's disease (29, 10, 10 days)	Hodgkin's disease (12, 7, 7, 7 days),
spinal injury (25 days),	parasitic disease (41 days),
cigarette smoking (10 days),	spinal meningitis (7 days),
schizophrenia (10,10, 10 days),	overactive thyroid (7 days),
	gout (7, 7, 8, 6 days),
	arteriosclerosis (14 days),
arthritis (10, 10, 10 days),	appendicitis (5 days),

enlarged prostate (10, 10 days)	acute lymphatic leukemia (14, 8, 12, 20 days),
cataracts (14 days),	anemia and lupus (14, 16, 26, 16, 14 days),
bronchitis (39 days),	
pneumonia (4 days),	muscular dystrophy (15, 8, 11 days),
typhoid fever (8 days),	
sterility (10 days),	chicken pox (4 days),
syphilis (16 days),	herpes (12 days),
uterine fibroid (28 days),	intestinal tapeworm (14 days),
Bright's disease (14 days),	
blindness in one eye (30 days),	menstrual problems (21 days),
malnutritional edema (40 days),	rheumatoid arthritis (22 days),
nasal polyps (24 days),	epilepsy (21 days),
gastric ulcer (19 days),	diabetes (7 days),
nymphomania (16 days),	chronic gastritis (29 days).
mental condition (insanity) (39 days),	

Dr. Shelton gives two studies in the appendix which can be summarized here to show the healing effect of fasting. (Book: *Fasting for the Health of It*)

b. Dr. Benesh & Dr. McEachen

In this study 714 cases were carefully supervised by Dr. Gerald Benesh, D.C., and Dr. James McEachen, D.C., from 1952-1958 in Escondido, California.[69]

Disease	Number of cases	Cases Remedied or Improved	Cases Not Helped
High blood pressure	141	141	0
Colitis	88	77	0
Sinusitis	67	64	3
Anemia	60	52	8
Hemorrhoids	51	48	3
Arthritis	47	39	8
Bronchitis	42	39	3
Kidney Disease	41	36	5
Benign Tumors	38	32	6
Heart Disease	33	29	4
Asthma	29	29	0
Ulcers	23	20	3
Hay Fever	19	17	2
Goiter	11	11	0
Pyorrhea	8	6	2
Gallstones	7	6	1
Cancer	5	5	0
Multiple Sclerosis	4	3	1
Total	741	654	60

c. Dr. Esser

Dr. William Esser, N.D., D.C., supervised 225 cases from 1945-1947 in Lake Worth, Florida.[70]

The following is the breakdown of those fasts.

Disease	Number of Cases	Cases Recovered	Cases Improved	Cases Not Helped
Dyspepsia	21	18	3	0
Pyorrhea	20	8	12	0
Asthma	19	16	0	3
Eczema	18	11	4	3
Benign Tumors	18	14	3	1
Insomnia	17	13	2	2
Ulcers	14	8	4	2
Diabetes	14	12	2	0
Kidney Disease	12	10	2	0
Sinusitis	12	9	3	0
Gallstones	11	6	5	0
Anemia	11	7	4	0
Gonorrhea	8	8	0	0
Poliomyelitis	8	6	2	0
Appendicitis	6	6	0	0
Epilepsy	5	3	2	0
Acne Vulgaris	5	3	2	0
Multiple Sclerosis	4	0	2	2
Tuberculosis	2	2	0	0
Total	225	160	52	13

These are very significant numbers showing statistical significance through water fasting.

d. Dr. Gross

In this study 447 cases were carefully supervised by Dr. Robert Gross, D.C., Ph.D., from 1957-1963 in Hyde Park, New York.[71]

Disease	Number of Cases	Cases Recovered	Cases Improved	Cases Not Helped
High Blood Pressure	54	38	16	0
Arthritis	42	28	10	4
Nasal Catarrh	39	36	2	2
Constipation	36	31	3	2
Hepatitis	36	34	2	0
Goiter	33	18	12	3
Psoriasis	32	18	10	4
Heart Disease	31	18	13	0
Mental Disorders	29	19	10	0
Bronchitis	24	22	1	1
Colitis	23	11	12	0
Hemorrhoids	23	18	5	0
Varicose Veins	23	20	2	1
Hay Fever	22	7	15	0
Total	447	318	113	17

The big question could be why the cases not helped, were not helped? Primarily because they needed to go on a strict vegan, or raw vegan diet for a long time, or there could be other complications besides what was mentioned. But the evidence is overwhelming for the number of people that recovered in each of these cases. A statistician could easily take these figures and show that it is statically significant!

To go into what types of problems were healed by what types and lengths of a fast is beyond the scope of this book. But just about any book you pick up on fasting that is by a medical person will give numerous examples of healings through fasting and diet. This book is written for the average person who wants to fast under 10 days and is not intended to deal with the problems mentioned above, which should be done under a physician's care.

e) Dr. Scott

Dr. David J. Scott has a degree as a Chiropractor, D.C., and went on for several other specialized degrees (Doctor of Medicine (overseas) and a Naturalopathic doctor ND). He was the founding president of the International Association of Hygienic Physicians and taught physiology at Great Lakes College. He was in practice for over 60 years and he water fasted under direct supervision some 20,000 patients.

Dr. Scott was unique in that he used the latest technologies to demonstrate the status of health by physiological parameters. Dr. Scott's office has a fully functional and modern scientific laboratory. From there he provides standardized testing to determine multiple indicators used to monitor a persons' progress during the fasting process. These extremely sensitive but standard medical technologies, including blood work, can discover early and even late signs of disease. He is the only one in the country that uses this kind of measurements during a long water fast.

"Many conditions may be uncovered through our testing. The many treating methods available frequently only relieve the symptoms. While utilizing these methods, in time one may move from acute disease into suppressed chronic disease. Left unhealed, the chronic disease in time may move from chronic inflammation into degeneration and even end in malignancy. By our methods we clearly document when your disease markers are brought into remission or healing.

If you go back to your old habits we most likely will find you are only beginning to refeed those same diseases again."

"The following are some of the many patients conditions benefited in over 50 years by therapeutic fasting:"

Acholasia	Constipation	Heart Disease	Prostate
Acid Reflux	Crohn's	Hemorrhoids	Disease
Acne Rosacea	Disease	Hiatal Hernia	Pruritus Ani
Acne Vulgaris	Cystitis	High	Psoriasis
Allergies	Depression	Cholesterol	Pulmonary
Anemia	Diabetes	Hyperacusis	Fibrosis
Angina Pectoris	Digestive	Hypertension	Pyorrhea
Arrhythmia	Disorders	(High Blood	Rectal Prolapse
Arteritis	Disc Herniation	Pressure)	Rheumatoid
Arthritis	Diverticulitis	Iritis	Arthritis
Asthma	Diverticulosis	Irritable Bowel	Sciatica
Atonic Bowel	Emphysema	Kidney Disease	Seizures
Blepharoptosis	Facial	Kidney Stones	(Epilepsy)
Blocked	Neuralgia	Liver Disease	Sinusitis
Arteries	Fevers	Macular	Sleep Apnea
Breast Cysts	Fibroids	Degeneration	Sleep Disorders
Breast Disease	Fibromyalgia	Migraine	Stroke
Bronchltls	Fistulac	Headaches	Disabilities
Bursitis	Fracture	Multiple	Tendonitis
Candidiasis	Healing Support	Sclerosis	Thrombo-
Catarract	Gall Bladder	Myositis	phlebitis
(early stage)	Disease	Nicotine	Tic Douloureux
Chemical	Gallstones	Addiction	Torticollis
Sensitivity	Gastritis	Ovarian Disease	Tumors
Cholecystitis	Glaucoma	Pancreatitis	(Benign)
Chronic Fatigue	(early stage)	Parotitis	Ulcers
Colitis	Goiter	Paroxysmal	Varicose Veins
Congestive	Gout	Tachycardia	and Ulcers
Heart Failure	Hay Fever	Polymyalgia	Vertigo
		Polymyositis	

A study on heart disease and diabetes is worth citing here. This study was done on people who did a one day a week fast and it showed that a one day fast a week can be biochemically beneficial, for heart patients and it can also be beneficial for diabetics. "People who fast seem to receive a

82

heart-protective benefit," said Benjamin D. Horne, Ph.D., M.P.H., study author and director of cardiovascular and genetic epidemiology at Intermountain Medical Center and adjunct assistant professor of biomedical informatics at the University of Utah in Salt Lake City. Researchers first examined the records of the Intermountain Heart Collaborative Study registry comprised of patients who had undergone coronary angiography, an X-ray examination of the blood vessels of the heart to look for blockages, between 1994 and 2002. Of those patients, 4,629 men and women, average age 64, could clearly be diagnosed either with coronary artery disease (CAD) -- which is at least 70 percent narrowing or blockage detected in at least one artery, or as free of significant CAD -- less than 10 percent narrowing or blockage.

Of this group, those who fasted were significantly less likely to be diagnosed with CAD (59 percent had 70 percent or greater blockage) than those who did not fast (67 percent had 70 percent or greater blockage). "Fasting was the strongest predictor of lower heart disease risk in the people we surveyed. Fasting was associated with lower odds of being diagnosed with CAD by 39 percent. When the researchers compared only those diagnosed with CAD with those who had minimal or no coronary disease (less than 10 percent blockage), the impact of fasting was even more striking, with the odds of a CAD diagnosis being lower by 45 percent.

Benjamin D. Horne, Ph.D., continues "When you abstain from food for 24 hours or so, it reduces the constant exposure of the body to foods and glucose," he said. "One of the major problems in the development of the metabolic syndrome and the pathway to diabetes is that the insulin-producing beta cells become desensitized. Routine fasting may allow them to resensitize -- to reset to a baseline level so they work better." The researchers looked separately at people with diabetes, who are not encouraged to skip meals, and found the same association of fasting and healthier arteries in both those with diabetes and those without diabetes.[72]

There are different types of cleansing diets and fasts that can be done with juices, such as an intestinal cleanse or a kidney cleanse, etc. Dr. Norman Walkers expertise was the colon cleanse and he was also an expert in these different cleanses thru fruits and juices. Colon cleanse is one type of a cleansing approach.

The Gerson diet uses diet and juicing. The Gerson Therapy uses a strict or raw vegetarian diet and about 13 glasses of freshly made juices a day. The Gerson Diet is one of the best healing diets for healing degenerative diseases like cancer and arthritis. The late Dr. Max Gerson is one of the key people in establishing diet therapy as a holistic practice.

There are some misconceptions about fasting from the scientific literature where studies on rats and studies in vitro (in a test tube or Petri dish) have shown that fasting is not healthy. So they apply these findings to humans and say that fasting is not healthy for humans. The fact that fasting is successfully used as a therapy for many types of illness proves that fasting is not only healthy but healing. Studies on animals have shown that fasting prolongs the life span of animals. Studies have shown that fasting decreases the incidence of infection and enhances immunoglobulin levels. Many studies could be discussed on fasting.

3. Paavo Airola Fasting Cancer Program

Paavo Airola, PhD, ND, in his booklet *Cancer Causes, Prevention and Treatment the Total Approach*, published in 1972 gives a good insight of cancer treatment before 1970 in Europe, and many of the methods are still valid today. The booklet was a paper delivered to the Ninth Annual Cancer Convention of the International Association of Cancer Victims and Friends.[73] Apparently, in Europe they have the same problems of suppression and persecution that is found in the U.S. since the opening sentence in his booklet he states: "First I want to make it perfectly clear* that I do not offer a cure for cancer." The asterisk/footnote states: *Mainly to protect myself against persecution, by over-zealous government agencies who, in the name of protecting the public, mercilessly attack anyone who not only dares to advise but even to report on unorthodox cancer therapies.

"There are several hundred so-called biological clinics in Europe, most of them directed by medical doctors, where drugless, biological medicine is practiced. In my book, *There is a Cure for Arthritis*, I list over a dozen such clinics with the complete addresses and names of the doctors. The most prominent cancer specialists in Germany using biological therapies in the treatment of cancer are Dr. Josef Issels, Prof. Werner Kollath and Prof. Lampert. However, there are over 4,000 medical doctors in Germany, members of the Association of Naturopathic (Biological) Doctors, who apply biological therapies in the treatment of most diseases, including cancer. All of my statements made about causes of cancer, and to effective nutritional and other biological methods of approaching cancer treatment, are well documented. Again, I do not offer a new or any other kind of cure for cancer - I report only what various cancer researchers have found and how cancer is successfully treated in European biological clinics. In this country, [America] all harmless, unorthodox treatments of cancer are outlawed leaving only surgery, radiation or chemotherapy. I feel that the millions of people who suffer from cancer are entitled to know the truth."

Following is Dr. Airola's section on using fasting for cancer or other degenerative diseases. This juice fasting approach as he indicates above is used in European biological clinics. Most American clinics utilize water fasting rather than juice fasting. A twenty-one day fast is considered normal for therapeutic fasting in Europe.

"One of the most important components of the total, combined anti-cancer program is the detoxification of the whole body. The underlying reason why the organism succumbs to cancer in the first place is the diminished or broken down resistance to the carcinogenic factors mainly due to the disordered metabolism, weakened activity of essential organs, such as liver, kidneys and pancreas, and general auto-toxemia. The purpose of juice fasting is to normalize all the vital body processes, revitalize the liver and other cleansing organs, cleanse the whole body of accumulated toxins, restore the digestive and assimilative functions of the stomach and intestinal tract, and, in general, increase the body's protective and healing capacity. The success of most anti-cancer programs in European biological clinics, as well as the Gerson's cancer therapy, or Dr. Kelly's program is attributed largely to their thorough cleansing programs."[74]

"Short, repeated cleansing fasts on raw vegetable and fruit juices are advisable. Most useful juices are red beet (from tops and roots),[75] carrot, green juice (made from leafy green vegetables, grape,[76] lemon, and all dark-colored juices. During fasting, daily coffee enemas are used - one cup of strong, freshly brewed coffee in a one pint of water, used as a retention enema - to stimulate the liver and increase its detoxifying activity. Although healthy persons can fast on their own, cancer patients should fast only under sympathetic professional supervision."[77]

Drinking juices allows the body to assimilate all of the vital substances in the quickest possible time. It may only take ten to fifteen minutes to assimilate juices properly made. However, it may take several hours to digest juice that is still in the pulp or liquefied stage (with solids). Juices give the cells in the body all the elements they need in a way that is easily assimilated.

4. The Breuss Cancer Cure through Juice Fasting

A man in Austria who was not medically trained named Rudolf Breuss started leading people in long juice fasts and many people were completely healed of cancer and other degenerative diseases. Later a fasting Institute was started in his name: Breuss Fasting Clinic Durhotel Chattenbuhl, Germany. Part three of the book goes into the cures of many other types of degenerative diseases through his juice fasting method. Rudolf Breuss is one of many doctors in Europe that use juice fasting as a method of healing. There is a company Biotta Naturals (a product of Switzerland, distributed by CAJ Food Products, Inc.[78]) promoting, *Breuss Vegetable Juice*, which is his formula. It tastes good but is expensive.

Rudolf Breuss Juice Mixture
"To prepare the juice, take 3/5 beets, 1/5 carrots, 1/5 celeriac (celery), and then add a little black radish and one egg-sized potato. For example:
- 300 g (9.6 oz.) beet root
- 100 g (3.2 oz.) carrots
- 100 g (3.2 oz.) celeriac (celery root)
- 30 g (1.06 oz.) black radish root
- 1 potato, the size of an egg

Note: It is not crucial to add the potato juice, except for the cancer of the liver where it is necessary.

Use a modern juice extractor, or press the vegetables the old-fashioned way, then put the juices through a tea strainer or a linen towel. There is a tablespoon of sediment for each quarter liter of juice, which must not be consumed.

This sediment would make the juice more difficult to drink and, more importantly, would serve as food for the cancer.

The cancer lives only on solid foods taken into the body. If for 42 days the patient only drinks vegetable juices and tea, the cancerous growth dies while the person can live through it all very well! It is better if a few days before starting this treatment, the patient drinks approximately one-quarter liter (1 cup/250 ml) of juice per day. The patient may go up to one half liter but this is not necessary.

Drink the juice slowly with the help of a spoon. Do not swallow it immediately but let the juice remain in the mouth for a few moments. Every now and again, the patient may have a mouthful of sauerkraut juice, which is beneficial to the patient. The juices are to be taken as indicated. A little lemon juice can be added but never apple juice! Freshly squeezed apple juice is allowed in between by itself but never mixed with the other juices. You may drink as much sage tea with St. John's Wort, peppermint and balm as you want, but do not add any sugar."[79]

"Over the years I have noticed that so-called failures of the treatment could be attributed to patients not following it in all aspects. An estimated 40,000 cancer patients and others suffering from seemingly incurable illnesses have regained their health through my juice treatment.

I beg you to remember how many great inventions were made by lay people. The most important thing, in the end, is the success of an idea and its usefulness for humankind. Scientists should acknowledge this fact, even if they cannot yet explain it. They should not care with whom or where the invention originated. I would be extremely happy if you could improve my Total Cancer Treatment even more by combining it with other successful methods of cancer therapy."[80]

A forward in the book by J. Rancout, MD (Lac Simon)[81] is worth noting. "As a medical doctor in Canada, I worked for many years in a special clinic for cancer patients. Everything in the clinic was geared toward making these patients as comfortable as possible until the day they died. It was called palliative care. . . .

"When I first read the book by Rudolf Breuss, which had been presented to me by my colleague, Dr. von Winterfeldt-Schubert, I realized that Breuss' fasting method was the simplest and most natural way possible to treat cancer. Breuss was a humble man whose only desire was to offer help and hope to a suffering people. He was so close to the laws of nature that he was able to develop an effective treatment for cancer. His very simplicity gave him an advantage over the complicated and mechanistic way in which medical treatment is often applied today.

"The Breuss Treatment is so effective because it deals with cancer and other chronic diseases by cleansing the whole system. The liquids used during the fast are rich in vitamins and minerals, keeping the body nourished; meanwhile, the metabolism is allowed to get back into balance; finally, a deep detoxification process eliminates whatever poisons, abnormalities and wastes are present in the body.

"A positive outcome of this treatment is closely tied to a person's attitude. People who go through with the six-week fast have a strong will and are convinced and determined that they will heal themselves with natural methods. Since attitude influences the whole metabolism, these people are truly taking their health into their own hands. The fast is often the beginning of a physical and spiritual awakening, compelling people to ensure their future health by turning their lives around, adopting positive habits and living closer to nature."[82]

VII. Detoxification Methods

"May the God of peace make you perfect and holy; and may you all be kept safe and blameless, spirit, soul and body, for the coming of our Lord Jesus Christ."

1 Thess 5.23.

In this section Jim gives his experience and research on these topics. This whole chapter on Detoxification Methods is not needed in most fasting situations but it can be beneficial and some knowledge of them is helpful. These detoxification methods are an aid to fasting.

1. Enemas and Purgatives

Dr. Airola states that enemas are given in all of the European health clinics that he knows of but that the number of enemas given differs. One Sanatorium gives enemas once every morning or every second morning. Another Institute gives enemas 2 to 3 times a day (morning, noon and evening). Some clinics give enemas twice a day. Dr. Airola recommends at least once a day in the morning. Then he recommends continuing the enema for two or three days after stopping the fast until the bowels start moving naturally and normal peristalsis is established. He does not recommend using enema's regularly or for prolonged periods, fasting is the exception.

Dr. Airola points out that; "The main purpose of fasting is to help the body to cleanse itself from accumulated toxic wastes. By the process of autolysis, a huge amount of morbid matter, dead cells and diseased tissues are burned; and the toxic wastes which have accumulated in the tissues for years, causing disease and premature aging, are loosened and expelled from the system. The alimentary canal, the digestive and eliminative system, is the main road by which these toxins are thrown out of the body. Since, during fasting, the natural bowel movements cease to take place, the toxic wastes would have no way of leaving the system, except with the help of enemas and colonics."[83]

Dr. Bragg who has fasted and supervised fasting for over seventy years, does not believe in enemas or purgatives. He states that; "Continued over a long period of time, it will set up irritation and wash out important internal and mucous membrane secretions and evacuate the bacteria necessary for good bowel function." He also states that the fast is a time of physiological rest and that the body has its own sanitation and antiseptic system within the bowels. "From time to time, during a fast, there may be some bowel elimination. But if there is none, you are not going to be poisoned."[84]

Dr. Bragg also writes; "I don't believe in an enema any time . . . I don't believe in forcing nature and the use of the enema, in my opinion, is most unnatural. This includes taking any kind of laxative before or during the fast. The bowel has its own sanitary and antiseptic machinery, and the residue that was in your bowel at the beginning of your fast will be neutralized until the fast is over. Nature's plumbing system is perfect if your will allow it to work naturally."[85]

Dr. Shelton also does not recommend enemas except in the case of someone with hemorrhoids or an emotionally upset faster who believes they need a bowel movement.

The author has done seven day juice fasts with no enema's and seven day juice fasts with many enemas'. I believe they do help, but I have not seen a big difference between using enemas or not using them. But I did see a big positive difference when I did a series of colonics during an eight day juice fast. I do encourage enemas and colonics during a fast since it is a time of physiological purification and these help, also it's a good learning experience.

These are helpful in the detoxification process but not necessary during a long fast since enemas and colonics can be done anytime. I do recommend that everyone does a series of colonics to get rid of any worms and parasites that may be living in the colon.

Colonics (colon therapy) are not necessary during a long fast and can be done at any time but they increase the detoxification process. For people that are seeking fasting for healing and major detoxification a colonic is recommended. As explained in the next section on colonics they are a major way to get rid of worms and parasites. About 20 to 30% of everyone in the U.S., who has never done colonics probably has parasites and worms in them. In underdeveloped countries like Africa it is probably 50 to 70% or more of the population has colon parasites and worms.

I recommend doing at least one or two enemas and if possible do three enemas, during a long 7 day juice fast. But it seems best to wait several days (perhaps two or three) before doing an enema and letting the bowel empty itself, the way it normally does. That way all the major solids will pass on their own without using an enema. Three or four days into the fast an enema will flush out the small solids and ill-smelling liquids in the intestines. The evening time, when you're at home undisturbed, seems to be a good time to do an enema.

In the "Starting a Long Fast" section I recommend using Prune Juice on the second morning of the fast to flush out the bowels. It could be best to wait a day or two after drinking prune juice and then do an enema on the third, fourth or fifth day. Solids take several days to leave the bowels.

But you may decide not to do an enema at all. It is helpful and highly recommended to do at least one enema during a fast, preferably two. But if you decide not to do an enema, then it would be best to drink a bottle of prune juice on the second, third or fourth day of the fast. The prune juice will help flush your system out and act as a purgative. It will have a similar effect as an enema but not as efficient.

There is no need to do an enema under three days. For one day fast or for a three day fast enemas are not needed but dong an enema or colonic during a fast is the best time to do it, greater cleansing. For four days or more an enema or colonics might be advisable.

2. Colon Therapy and Parasites

"As for this kind, it is cast out only by prayer and fasting." Mt 17:21; Mk 9.29

Colon Therapy or Colonics are in some ways better then enemas because they accomplish a lot more. An enema goes in as far as the sigmoid flexor in the colon and it could go to the splenic flexure, which is the descending part of the colon. A colonic does the descending, the traverse and the ascending part of the colon all the way to the ileo cecal value (to the small intestine). But enemas can and do accomplish a lot.

In order to do the whole descending colon with an enema you would have to raise your feet above your waist or do a head stand. Also an enema has limited pressure and temperature control and requires effort on your part. Whereas in a colonic the operator controls the flow of water in and out, the pressure and temperature of the water. You lay there relaxed first, on your side and then on your back while the operator does all the work.

The colonic has a clear tube going from your anus to the colonic machine. The operator can watch what comes out and one part of the tube goes through the machine in a clear tube with a light and the operator can stop and catch something if needed. Thus they know when a worm comes out.

Colonics are bigger in Europe then America. In Germany only Doctors are allowed to do colonics, it is a basic part of their medical practice. In the U.S. some doctors and even some naturopathic doctors are against colonics, these have probably never done colonics themselves.

Dr. Walker M.D. highly recommends enemas and colonics as a regular part of one's lifestyle. "Let us be frank and honest about it: No one man has all the answers. Nevertheless, the very Best of Diets can be no better than the Very Worst, if the sewage system, the eliminative organs in your anatomy, is clogged up with a collection of waste and corruption. This is one particular angle of the problem of nutrition which is generally overlooked. I refer to the elimination from the system of waste matter from the colon."[86]

He goes on to point out that most foods eaten in home and restaurants are not efficient in colon cleansing. Coating builds up on the inner walls of the colon like plaster on a wall. As this coating thickens less nutrients are absorbed. The fiber that should do some housecleaning on the walls of the colon does not clean because the food is cooked and the fiber does not work as well, if at all. "Instead of furnishing nourishment to the nerves and muscles, cells and tissues of the walls of the colon, cooked foods actually cause starvation of the colon. A starved colon may let a lot of fecal matter pass through it, but it is unable to carry on the last of the digestive and nourishing processes and functions intended for it.

"If I had seen only a few colonic irrigations give successful results, I would be justified in withholding my judgment in regard to their efficacy. Having seen literally thousands of them, all giving results with no laxative or cathartic could give, I must admit that I am dumbfounded whenever anyone questions their value or efficacy. As a

94

matter of fact long ago I arrived at the conclusion that no treatment of any ailment, sickness or disease could be effective unless and until the waste matter had been washed out of the colon by means of colonic irrigations, if available, or enemas if they were not available."[87]

Oftentimes experts give the argument that animals don't do enemas but Dr. Walker gives an example: "As a matter of fact, I have seen herons and other similar birds in Florida stand by a river or pool of water, fill their long beaks, and inject water into the rectum in order to give themselves an enema or colon irrigation. I never asked these birds what school, college or university they attended or who taught them this principle of internal lavage."[88]

Dr. Walker M.D. gives his opinion on having a cleansing program. "It took many years to accumulate whatever corruption that has adhered to the inside walls of your colon; therefore, give the irrigations that chance to cleanse you thoroughly. Thereafter, I am convinced that about twice a year, throughout life, a series of six colon irrigations should help Nature keep the body healthy. Bear in mind that colon irrigations are less expensive than hospitalization and surgeon's fees, and more certain of beneficial results!"[89]

Dr. Bernard Jensen, a chiropractor and nutritionists is a well known leader in the field of health. He emphasizes the need for Bowel care with enemas and colonics. "I believe that the number-one source of the misery and decay we are witnessing in our society today is autointoxication - self-poisoning caused by microorganisms, metabolic waste, and other toxins in the body. Through autointoxication, the human body becomes the unwitting host of uncleanliness with its entourage of imbalance, derangements, perversions, sickness, and disease."[90]

Dr. Jensen gives some good insight into the process of cleansing toxins and poisons. "Tissue laced with internal

95

(metabolic) toxins or external toxins (from polluted air or water, or tobacco smoke) can't assimilate nutrients well or eliminate its own wastes efficiently. If injured, toxin-laced tissues heal extremely slowly until they are cleansed of those toxins. The bowel is the source of most internal toxic material, which makes its way into the blood and lymph through the bowel wall and is then carried to and deposited in the tissues. A cleaner bowel leads to cleaner blood, which leads to cleaner tissues, which then rebuild more easily."[91]

Dr. Jensen points out those doctors do not do a good job of saving themselves from colon death. "According to statistics compiled by the Registrar General of England, no group has contributed more to the death rate from intestinal diseases than doctors. These statistics show that the death rate of doctors is higher than those of both agricultural workers and the English population in general."[92] Of course most doctors do not believe in the need for colon therapy. Dr. Jensen emphasizes the use of colema board for doing enemas.

The intestinal walls are semi-permeable and one of the largest detoxification organs in the body. Doing colonics during a fast is a way of hurrying the detoxification process. During a colonic the body is releasing toxins and mucus and slug that are packed into the walls of the colon. It can also flush out cancer cells and other diseases that may be forming in the colon.

Stanley Weinberger (an expert in this field) gives a good explanation of some of the benefits of colon therapy. "Colon therapy has an antiseptic and solvent actions on the intestines, whereby putrefactive material, impacted fecal matter, excess mucous, and even pus and infected tissue are removed from the colon. This leaves a cleaner, healthier colon, which means a healthier body.

"Colon therapy increases the water level and diuretic action of the body. Water is absorbed into the body, which increases the volume of the blood. Circulation is thereby increased, resulting in greater bathing of the individual cells, thus diluting toxins and flushing them out; relieving uremia and toxemia; and increasing elimination both through kidneys and skin as well as the bowel. All this generally assists the cardiovascular and circulatory systems' efficiency.

"Colon therapy with oxygen has an anthelmintic action; that is, parasites are removed. Many patients are found to have some form of parasites, the most common being tapeworm. Various other types found are hookworms, pinworms, roundworms, whipworms, and many other exotic forms. Sources of tapeworms are usually beef, pork or fish. Many vegetarians also are infected with various parasites by easting vegetables or fruit infested with parasite eggs. Dr. Norman Walker said: 'Experience has taught me that no health and healing procedures can be as successful as those which have a series of colon irrigations as the prelude to any health treatment.'"[93]

"The two major factors that make an epidemic of parasites possible are: 1) lack of sanitation, and 2) colons which are clogged and impacted from years of improper eating habits, providing a warm and well-fed breeding ground for worms and parasites to proliferate.

"The multitude of different symptoms caused by parasites can be baffling to many doctors, who receive little training in diagnosing and treating parasitic infections. Unless people have major symptoms, doctors often mis-diagnose cases as bacterial infections, but unfortunately, antibiotics have no effect on most parasites.

"Colon cleansing (colonics) can go a long way toward eliminating parasites and accumulated, impacted wastes in the large intestine. These wastes can be caused by eating the wrong kinds of foods, emotional distress, and weak muscle tone of the colon. Removal of these wastes by colon cleansing - wherein the colon is flushed with filtered water

97

through a series of fills and releases - results in a renewed sense of health, vitality and energy in the individual's entire system."[94]

"One of every four people in the world is infected by roundworms, which cause fever, cough, and intestinal problems. A quarter of the world's people have hookworms, which can cause anemia and abdominal pain. A Third of a billion people suffer from the abdominal pain and diarrhea caused by whipworms."[95]

In 1976 a nationwide study of over four hundred and fourteen thousand samples of feces indicated that one in every six people has one or more parasites living somewhere in his or her body. Dr. Juranek the assistant chief of the Centers for Disease Control in Atlanta said, "I'm sure that this high infection rate comes as a surprise to those who never considered parasitic diseases to be a major problem in the U.S."[96]

The rate of infection is actually higher since parasites and worms do not always show up in every stool sample. Cathie K. a colonic therapists of over ten years said that many of her patients, when they first come to have a colonic done, have worms. And most of her clients are health conscious. She pointed out that only one out of twelve stool samples will show parasites, so doctor's tests on stool samples often miss the presence of parasites.

Dr. Louis Parrish, M.D. writes of infections of intestinal protozoa[2] and that "among 300 million U.S. inhabitants, I feel confident in estimating that 7 million people are infected." "Amoebiasis and Giardiasis are only recently being recognized as a forgotten cause of long-term illness in millions of Americans. The allopathic medical community has by undefinable social and scientific attitudes

---

[2] Entamoeba histolytica, Giardia lamblia.

perfunctorily rejected these illnesses and to frequently accepted false negative lab results as a fact.

"The wide variety of gastrointestinal symptoms, fatigue and general toxicity can compromise a clinical picture and make these infections hard to diagnose. The few drugs available to treat protozoa infections can have intolerable side effects and often do not eradicate the pathogens."[97]

"Candida Albicans is yeast that lives in the mouth, throat, intestines, and genitourinary tract of most humans. Candida is usually considered to be a normal part of the bowel flora (organisms that coexist in our lower digestive tract). A healthy immune system normally keeps Candida under control, but when the immune system is weakened, the natural balance between the human host and the Candida is altered. Unless the body's defenses are given some assistance, colonies of Candida will flourish throughout the body producing many adverse physical and mental symptoms collectively known as candidiasis."[98]

An experienced colon therapists Cathie says it takes between five to fifteen sessions to totally clean out the colon. This could be done grouped together or once a week. This depends on the age and dietary patterns of the person. Some people come in once a year, others several times a year for colon therapy, but to do several at a time might be the best approach.

And the number of colonics needed could also depend on what they are holding onto emotionally. There is one author who suggests that some of our emotions get tied into the food we eat which also is attached to the feces matter stuck to the sides of the colon, which a colonics washes out.

One author points out that, "Once worms or parasites are established in the body, these invaders do four things: 1. Worms can cause physical trauma to the body by perforation of the intestines, the circulatory system, the lungs, the liver

99

and so on... 2. Worms can also erode, damage or block certain organs. They can lump themselves together and make a ball, a tumor so to speak... 3. Parasites have to eat, so they rob us of our nutrients. They like to take the best of our vitamins and amino acids and leave the rest to us... 4. The last and most important way these scavengers cause damage is by poisoning us with their toxic waste. Each worm gives off certain metabolic waste products that our already weakened bodies have trouble disposing of.

"When the body is in an alkaline condition the parasitic infection sets in. It is best to keep the diet slightly acidic both as a preventive measure and when treating the infection. Foods that help keep the intestines acidic are apple cider vinegar and cranberry juice."[99] Garlic may also be another beneficial food.

Some signs of parasites can be: chronic fatigue; immune dysfunction; constipation; diarrhea; gas and bloating; anemia; nervousness; allergies. Some common parasitic diseases are: elephantiasis infestation by carrier mosquitoes; trichinosis infestation from undercooked meat; schistosomiasis infestation is through skin from infested fresh water; amebiasis infection from contaminated water and vegetables; sleeping sickness infestation from tsetse fly; malaria infested from female mosquitoes; roundworm infestation from food and/or water; diarrhea infected from vegetables and water; dwarf tapeworm infestation from contaminated water; and the pinworm infestation from food and/or water. Dogs, cats and other pets can also carry parasites.

Dr. Walker gives numerous examples of people that were sick some chronically ill that had a series of colonics done and they were healed. It was in many of these worms and parasites came out during the colonic.

Thus a major reason for doing a colonic is worms and parasites that end up in the colon. Worms are parasites that can be divided into roundworms (tapeworms, flukes) and flatworms (threadworms, pinworms, flatworms). Several common flukes are intestinal fluke; liver fluke; pancreatic flute. Most of these can be found in the colon and a colonic will kill them and flush them out.

Dr. Hulda Clark Ph.D., N.D. has some findings in her practice. "No matter how long and confusing is the list of symptoms a person has, from chronic fatigue to infertility to mental problems, I am sure to find only two things wrong: they have in them pollutants and/or **parasites**. I never find lack of exercise, vitamin deficiencies, hormone levels or anything else to be a primary causative factor."[100]

"Fasciolopsis buskii is the fluke (flatworm) that I find in every case of cancer, HIV infection, Alzheimer's, Crohn's disease, Kaposi's endometriosis, and in many people without these diseases."[101]

"The lower abdomen on the left side has the sigmoid colon as it comes down and bends. This is a favorite location for larger parasites to settle permanently. Flukes, roundworms, parasites of all kinds and their attentive bacteria and viruses can be felt if they produce gas and pain. Sometimes they live perfectly quietly, seemingly in harmony with us."[102]

Doing colonics during a fast speeds up the detoxification process. The author has done colonics during a fast and found colonics to be much easier and more efficient then an enema. The drawback is that an enema you can do by yourself in your bathroom but a colonics takes a scheduled session with a colonics therapists and costs money. But the money (average $50-75 per session) is well worth it, for the benefit it derives. Usually it is necessary to start with at least two sessions. If you're serious about house cleaning then it would be recommended to do three to nine colonics during a long fast. But having a colonic done can be done at any time and you do not need to be on a fast, but a fast will yield the best results.

3. How to do an Enema

A brief description of how to do an enema will be helpful here since some are not familiar with it. The first big obstacle will be the psychological one, some people make a big deal out of it, and others just do it.

First fill the water bottle (or enema bottle) up with lukewarm (body temperature water) and lubricate the end of the tube with a Vaseline, jelly or mineral oil. And it is also helpful to lubricate your annual canal a little too. 'Annusol' is a hemorrhoidal ointment for temporary relief of dryness and it has active ingredients for germs. This might be a better choice because of the active ingredients.

Some water may come out so put a towel on the floor. Hang the water-bottle up high (3 to 5 feet) so that it can flow down into you easily and have sufficient pressure. There are three or four positions that can be used in doing an enema. Kneeling down on the towel and put your head on the floor is one position. A second position is to lay on your right side with your legs folded up halfway. A third position is to lie on your back with your feet on the floor, when doing the enema. If you lay on your back you can push your hips up off the floor which will allow the water to enter easier. Laying on your right side is probably the easiest of the three positions.

You can try all three positions and see which works best, which means you'd have to do at least three enemas. Another possibility is to sit on the toilet and insert the tip but this is a bit more difficult to hold the water in, laying on your side, your back or your knees is be better.

Make sure the air is let out of the tube before inserting into your anus. Gently, slide in the lubricated tube into your anus. Open the value/clamp so that the water can flow freely into your bowl. Let some water flow in, clamp the value stopping it to allow your system to adjust to the water, open the value and continue. Let as much flow in until it feels a little uncomfortable then stop, wait a minute and continue.

At first you will feel some pressure in the rectal area and the water will want to come back out. Stop the water for a minute and let the water seep into your intestines. You may hear some groaning and movement into your intestines as the water enters in. Open the value/clip again and let the water flow in again, you may have to do this several times. If you feel some pain or discomfort stop the water running in and wait a minute, relax, breath. Try to empty the whole water bottle or most of it into your intestines.

It is best to try and retain the water for a few minutes before letting it out. Stand up or lie on your back and perhaps massage your stomach area to help loosen debris that may be stuck to your intestines. Or try doing some simple yoga exercises briefly, such as putting your feet into the air (an inversion). But any movement may release the spinster muscle at the anus and let water start to flow out.

Try to keep the water in for a few minutes before sitting on the toilet and allowing the water to flow out. Then just sit on the toilet and let the bowels empty out. Sitting could take fifteen minutes to a half hour or more so have some reading material nearby to help you relax.

The first time you do an enema you may have to do one and a half enemas. Because there are solids still in your rectum, the water may back up quickly and you may not be able to empty a whole water bottle into yourself. So just empty out that first attempt on the toilet and then start with a whole new bottle and do it again.

When doing an enema if you don't succeed the first time then try again later that day or the next day. You may want to fill the water bottle up again and add more water into your system. This will force the water up further into the intestinal tract providing a deeper cleansing. And if you don't get all the water from one bottle into you because you have to immediately have to sit on the toilet that is O.K. too. Practice and experience will help in the long run. Of course you will want to take a shower after doing an enema.

It might be advisable to wear two pairs of underwear and bring an extra pair to work with you. Sometimes the water in the colon may not come down for several hours. It may feel like you need to fart and a little water may come out, messing up your underwear. Wearing two pairs will help stop it touching your pants or skit, and the extra pair is for you to change with.

For a coffee enema you will want to retain the enema for ten to fifteen minutes thus laying quietly is best to hold it longer. Lie quietly, relax and try some deep or controlled breathing.

The question might be asked are enema's harmful? No they are not, an enema is safe but it may be a little uncomfortable, a little painful or even repulsive.

A religious practice that might help here: A good practice for personal protection before doing an enema (or any potentially harmful or fearful situation) is to plead the blood of Jesus. Make the sign of the cross three times and cover yourself three times with the precious blood of Jesus. Thus pray to cover yourself with the precious Blood of Jesus before doing an enema.

If you have some concerns, it could help to cover oneself with the blood of Jesus three times: one for external influences in the environment, one for physical influences on the body and one for internal influences in the soul (the mind, emotions and will). Here is a simple prayer, based on this principle of covering oneself with the Precious Blood of Jesus three times.

"I cover myself with the Precious Blood of Jesus in the name of the Father, of the Son and of the Holy Spirit. (Make the sign of the cross) I cover this bathroom and everything in it with the Precious Blood of Jesus, I cover my body and internal organs with the Precious Blood of Jesus and I cover my thoughts, emotions and will with the Precious Blood of Jesus, Thank you Lord Jesus for your Precious Blood. Amen."

This formula of covering oneself with the precious blood of Jesus three times could be used at other times when you feel the need for the Lord's protection.

"Finally, draw your strength from the Lord and his mighty power. Put on the armor of God so that you may be able to stand firm against the tactics of the devil. Our battle is not against flesh and blood..." Eph 6.10-12

4. Coffee Enemas

The coffee enema is part of the Gerson Therapy routine and has become a routine enema for detoxification of the liver, used by many people. The purpose of coffee enemas is to lower serum toxins via. the colon. It pulls the toxins and poisons out of the liver into the colon, which get expelled.

The way to give a coffee enema is the same way to give a regular enema except that you want to hold the enema in longer, for 12-15 minutes. By holding the enema in allows more of it to be absorbed in the colon and to do its work. By absorbing more will allow it to have a better cleanse of the kidneys from toxins.

The way to prepare the coffee enema is to add 3 tablespoons of drip-grind organic coffee to a quart of boiling water for three minutes. Simmer it for 15 minutes then allow it to cool to body temperature. Make sure you strain it to get out all the coffee grins. Have some coffee filters available and strain the coffee through them. You only need to put about 8 ounces up the colon since more could be absorbed in the colon.

Drinking coffee does not have the same effect as a coffee enema. "Practitioners and patients who have had experience with coffee enemas, however, know that they are far more than a means of introducing stimulating caffeine into the bloodstream. From the patient's point of view, the coffee enema means relief from depression, confusion, general nervous tension, many allergy related symptoms and, most importantly, relief from severe pain."[103]

The theory behind the coffee enema is complicated but to give a brief explanation. The editors of Physiological Chemistry and Physics in discussing the use of coffee enemas with cancer stated: "Caffeine enemas cause dilation of bile ducts, which facilitates excretion of toxic cancer breakdown products by the liver and dialysis of toxic products from blood across the colonic wall."[104]

"As a medication, the coffee enema is in a class by itself. While other agents classed as choleretics do increase bile flow from the liver, they do little to enhance detoxifying enzyme systems, and they do not ensure the passage of bile from the intestines out the rectum. Bile is normally reabsorbed up to 9 or 10 times before working its way out the intestines in feces. The enzyme enhancing ability of the coffee enema is unique among choleretics. Because it does not allow reabsorption of toxic bile by the liver across the gut wall, it is an entirely effective means of detoxifying the blood stream through existing enzyme systems in the liver and small bowel. Because clinical practice has shown coffee enemas to be well tolerated by patients when used as frequently as every four hours, the coffee enema may be classed as the only non-reabsorbed, effective, repeatable choleretic in the medical literature.

"The contribution of low serum toxin levels by regular administration of coffee enemas is basic to increased cell energy production; enhanced tissue integrity, improved circulation, improved immunity, and improved tissue repair and regeneration which have been observed clinically to result from the administration of the combined regime of Gerson."[105]

The coffee enemas help to detoxify the liver and intestines of carcinogens and noxious chemicals. The coffee is boiled, strained, then decanted through a mesh strainer but not filtered. Research indicates that glutathione-S-transferase, the body's most powerful enzyme system and central to the anticancer defense, does not respond to filtered coffee since the filtering removes key chemicals called palmitates which stimulate glutathione's detoxifying activities.

The coffee enema should be used at body temperature. If the solution is slightly warm to touch (not hot or cold), it is going to be more comfortable to hold in longer. Experiments have shown that the caffeine is absorbed from the solution in about 12 minutes. Lay on your left side.

5. Dry Brushing

Body impurities and wastes are eliminated through the skin thus it is good to take showers every day. It is also good to keep warm since this conserves energy and can help elimination, chilling checks elimination.

Dr. Airola recommends doing a dry brush massage with a long handle natural bristle brush. He suggests doing it morning and evening during a fast for five to fifteen minutes. Using a brush make rotating motions to massage every part of your body. "You skin is your largest eliminative organ. Hundreds of thousands of tiny sweat glands act not only as the regulators of body temperature, but also as small kidneys, the detoxifying organs which are ready to cleanse the blood and free the system from health-threatening poisons."[106]

Dr. Airola lists the benefits of a dry brush massage. 1. It will effectively remove the dead layers of the skin and other impurities, and keep pores open. 2. It will stimulate and increase blood circulation. 3. It will stimulate hormone and oil-producing glands. 4. It stimulates nerve endings in the skin. 5. It will rejuvenate the complexion.[107]

The dry brush massages, will brush off any excretions given off through the skin and open up the skin pours. The skin provides easy access to the nervous and endocrine system. Dry brushing stimulates the glands, promoting their return to a proper function. The skin is the largest eliminative organ in the body. The skin needs to breathe and to be able to eliminate waste. Dry brushing stimulates and invigorates the nervous system and the glands and relieves stress and muscle tightness. It stimulates the acupressure points. It stimulates the eliminative capacity of the skin helping to release toxins. The skin will become rosy, resilient and youthful and clean.

Dry brushing stimulates hormone and oil producing glands as with the endocrine system. The endocrine system includes the pineal gland, pituitary gland, thyroid and parathyroid glands, thymus, adrenal, pancreas and islets of Langerhans, testes (male) and ovaries (female). These glands secrete and generate hormones that go directly into the blood and are used to regulate different parts of the body.

If the skin is real dry an oil massage may help such as with sesame, avocado, almond or extra virgin olive oil, cocoa butter or coconut oil works good. These cold pressed natural oils are good as a moisturizer.

Dry brushing is best done before taking a shower and done nude, mornings are a good time. Always begin brushing gently and don't overdo it. After a couple of weeks it will become natural, enjoyable and relaxing.

Do not brush if you have poison ivy, skin rashes, infections, or other skin problems, or inflammatory circulatory problems such as phlebitis.

It only takes about 5 to 10 minutes to do a dry brush massage depending on how many times and how fast you do it. You can start with your limbs, your hands or feet. If you start with your hands do the hands and arms then move to doing the feet and legs. A quick one would be 3 or 5 times and 7 for a little longer brush. In a circular motion make five circles on your arm top and bottom. The shape of the arm and the leg may take three sides for each, thus once on the right side of the leg and then left side and then the back of the same leg.

Then do the hips and butt, next the stomach area and chest, sides of body and then the lower back and upper back. Then do the shoulders and the back of the neck. Gently do the neck and parts of the face if it's comfortable.

What you need is a brush about the size of your hand with moderately soft natural vegetable fiber bristle. Synthetic or nylon may be too sharp and may hurt the skin. Every week or two wash the brush to get rid of impurities that may collect. It would be best if family members each had their own brush for hygienic reasons.

The skin sensitivity will vary from person to person and different parts of the body are more sensitive than other parts so brush gently at first. After a few days the skin starts to get used to the brushing and it will be easier. The dry brushing will tone and tighten the skin and also get rid of any troublesome cellulite, fatty deposits that get released through the skin.

Dry brushing gives a sense of well being; it is uplifting and feels great. The body is invigorated and the skin feels good. The skin gets a warm rosy glow and you feel your circulation stimulated and oxygen is increased through the pores. It is a difficult experience to describe, it is best understood if you just take and do dry brushing for a week or two, then you'll know.

6. Showers and Reflexology

Dr. Airola also recommends taking a hot-and-cold shower. Taking shower is, of course, necessary but whether the hot-and-cold shower routine is helpful you will have to decide. Try and experiment and do not take a shower for two days. You will notice a buildup of excretions on your skin but you would probably notice this even if you were not fasting.

Dr. Herbert Shelton does not recommend hot-cold showers since they might be a stress factor and do not increase stimulation of elimination. He also cautions against sunbathing for too long a period of time during a fast. And he states that "Sweat baths remove water from the fluids and tissues of the body - they remove nothing else."[108]

Reflexology can be helpful. All the energy centers from the organs in the body go out to the hands and feet (and also to the eyes, tongue, ears and other parts). It can be related to acupuncture and other massage techniques. All the different organs of the body are laid out on the bottom of the foot and by pressing on each pressure point it influences that particular organ. Reflexology is well accepted by health food and healing community.

Foot and hand reflexology are based on Zone Therapy, that there are ten energy currents - five on each half of the body - between the head and ten toes and fingers. Within these zones are the organs and muscles of the body.

"When the energy currents that flow through longitudinal zones build up at certain points, they create an accumulation of energy, or blockage, at those points. Referred to as energy blocks, they interrupt the smooth flow of energy throughout the body, causing the pain, disorder, disease or whatever problems which require healing."[109]

Acupuncture and Polarity Therapy are also based on the flow of energy currents in the body but these have different approaches in dealing with the energy zones. These therapies are much more complex and require professional training. Reflexology is very simple and straightforward and almost anyone can learn how to do it.

At least once or twice during a fast, massage the bottom of your feet. Start with each of your toes and go over your each foot to the base of your heel. Use the tips of your fingers to push into the skin and move your finger in a circle as you move along. There will be pressure points that hurt, that is good, massage it longer on that point and then move along. The pressure points that hurt are usually organs that are sensitive or hurting for some reason. Massaging those sore points will help release and circulate energy to that part of the body. After finishing pressing the whole foot with your finger, stroke it a few times to relax it. Do both feet.

Fasting works more on a cellular biological level rather than with the subtle energy currents of the body. But by doing reflexology during a long fast it can stimulate the organs and muscles and possibly help them to release toxins and poisons into the body to be eliminated.

7. Your Tongue and your Weight

Paul Bragg states; "Your tongue is a 'Magic Mirror'. Your tongue can reveal how much toxic material is stored in the cells and vital organs of your body....A few days of fasting will coat the tongue with a thick, white, rancid, toxic material that has a terrible odor. This heavy coating of toxic material can be scraped off and examined. In a fast, you can scrape the tongue clean, but in a few hours, the heavy toxic coating will return."[110]

This is an interesting phenomenon to observe. The tongue will become coated with a white liquid substance that it excretes. As the fast continues the tongue will start to become more its normal reddish color, starting from the tip and moving backwards, and the white coat will disappear. Usually there is not a real change in the tongue until the fifth or sixth day.

On a long 7-10 day fast I have seen this white coat slowly move backwards to about the middle of the tongue. And then on a long fast I have seen the tongue coated and not clear up at all but remain with its white coat. That is supposed to mean that the fast should continue but not always. It is interesting to note but I am not sure of its practical value in working with a fast. Thus, when you go on a long fast stick your tongue out and look in the mirror every day, if you want to. It may help to be used it as one of the means of determining when you should break the fast.

Weight yourself on the first day of the fast and on the last day of the fast. You will lose some weight, usually it is not that much, but everyone is different. I think you will lose a lot more weight on a water fast then on a juice fast. I lose between five and ten pounds on a seven day juice fast but I usually gain it back after eating again.

VIII. Extending Lifespan with Fasting

"Jehoshaphat was alarmed and resolved to have
recourse to Yahweh; he proclaimed a fast for all Judah."
2 Ch 20:3

1. Methods of extending lifespan

The question needs to be asked, what are the only
consistently proven methods of extending lifespan? A brief
review of the literature shows that there are four aspects that
extend life, giving a long healthy life, for the majority of
cases of longevity: 1. Vegetarian diet or very low protein
diet; 2. Moderation in the quantity of food (low calorie
intake); 3. Inner Calm (rejoices in virtue, rejects vice);
4. Fasting (inner cleansing).

In the US for 2011 the average life expectancy is
78.37 years and ranks #50 in the world. Twenty nine
countries have a life expectancy of 80 years or higher, the
highest average is 90 years old. This is according to the CIA
(Central Intelligence Agency) in August 2011. Research
from the older Adventist Mortality Study's (1958, 1960-
1965) showed that Adventist men (Adventist emphasize a
vegetarian diet) lived about 6.2 years longer, later analysis
showed 7.3 year longer life-expectancy average for men, for
women it was 4.4 years longer of life.[111]

A plant-based author Ross Horne a noted health
author pointed out that, "The longest-lived populations in the
world are accepted generally to be the people of Hunza in
northern Pakistan, Vilcabamba in Ecuador, and Georgia in
Russia. An analysis of these peoples living habits was
carried out under the auspices of the National Geographic in
1971 by Dr. Alexander Leaf [chief of medical services at
Massachusetts General Hospital in Boston] provided a good
reason why they outlived people of the Western world. The
traditional diets of these long-lived (by our standards) people

contained only half to two thirds the calories of the average American intake, about a quarter the amount of fat and half the protein. Their carbohydrate intake was about the same but was unprocessed instead of processed. As well, these people got more outdoor exercise and were less subject to stress than Americans."[112]

Dr. Airola relates from the same research: "Dr. Alexander Leaf, chief of medical services at Massachusetts General Hospital in Boston, made an extensive study in three sections of the world where people live extraordinarily long lives: The Andean village of Vilcabamba, Ecuador; the Hunza Kingdom in Kashmir; and the Black Sea coastal area of Abkhazia, in Russia."

"According to Dr. Alexander Leaf, M.D. who visited the Hunza and made an extensive study of their diet as related to their exceptionally long life, the factors mostly responsible for their long life are: 1) their total low-calorie diet (an average of 1900 calories a day) and 2) their predominantly vegetarian diet (only 1 percent of their protein intake come from animal sources). **Dr. Leaf says: 'I returned from my travels and convinced that vigorous, active old age, free from debility and senility, is possible.**"[113]

Dr. Paavo Airola describes centenarians in his book (1974); a Turkish man who was a vegetarian and has never eaten meat in his life. He walks a mile and a half every day and still works in an orchard. Shirali Mislimov tells his secret of a long life: "I was never in a hurry in my life, and I=m in no hurry to die now. There are two sources of long life: One is a gift of nature, and it is the pure air and clear water of mountains, the fruit of the earth, peace, rest, and the soft warm climate of the highlands. The second source is within us. He lives long who enjoys life and who bears no jealousy of others, whose heart harbors no malice or anger, who sings a lot and cries a little, who rises and retires with the sun, who likes to work, and who knows how to rest."[114]

Dr. Paavo Airola explains that a high protein diet is a sure road to premature aging. AThe Hunza example illustrates clearly that *it is not a high-protein, but a low-protein diet which has the greatest potential for optimum health and long life.* Their average daily intake of protein is about 30 grams. Many other long-living people in the world, like the Russians, Yukatan Indians, Todas, Abhkazians, Vilcabamba inhabitants, and Bulgarians, are people who eat low-protein diets. Hunzakuts eat meat once a month, at the most. According to a recent study of Dr. S. Magsood Ali, of Pakistan, only 1 percent of the Hunzakuts' protein intake was from animal sources. Bulgarians eat very little meat - perhaps 15 - 20 percent of the average Americans consumption. In Russia, only 12 percent of the total population is vegetarians, while 9 percent of all people who reach 100 years are vegetarians. The healthiest people in Latin America, with the longest life expectancy, are the Yucatan Indians, who never eat meat. Vilcabamba inhabitants in Ecuador show the largest number of centenarians of any place in the world - 1098 for every 100,000 people! According to Dr. Alexander Leaf, M.D., their average protein intake is 35-38 grams a day, and the total caloric intake is only 1200 to 1360 a day. They are almost 100 percent vegetarians."[115]

Another factor to be known about long life is that an inner peace is usually associated with long life. The negative passions of the soul do influence the body. Dr. Airola notes the longest known life span of a person in modern times: "The renowned Chinese scholar and herbalist, Professor Li Chung Yun, who lived to be 265 years of age. Don=t laugh! Professor Li Chung Yun's age is well documented. Being a world-famous scholar, he was in the public eye for over 200 years. At the age of 100, he was awarded by the Chinese government a special Honor Citation for extraordinary services to his country. This document is available in existing archives. For over 150 years after the award, the Professor was visited by countless Western scholars and students. It is reported that he gave a series of 28 lectures at the University of Sinkiang when he was over 200 years old.

"His life spanned four centuries - 16th, 17th, 18th, and 19th. He enjoyed excellent health, outlived 23 wives, and kept his own natural teeth and hair. Those who saw him at the age of 200 testified that he did not appear much older than a man in his fifties. Professor Li Chung Yun attributed his longevity to his life-long vegetarian diet and the regular use of rejuvenating herbs plus - may I add, an important plus - to his 'inward calm.' He used gotu-kola (hydrocotyle asiatica minor) and ginseng daily in the form of tea.

"Researchers and writers who studied his life in detail, attributed his long life to his vegetarian diet and special rejuvenative herb teas which he drank all of his life: ginseng and got-kola. Li Chung Yun himself, however, had a different idea for the reason of his long life. When asked to what he attributed his long life, he said: 'I attribute my long life to INWARD CALM.'

"In all my studies of people who lived extraordinarily long lives in various parts of the world, I have found that in addition to all the other factors, such as sound nutrition of simple, unadulterated foods, scanty eating, poison free environment, and plenty of exercise, they all possessed that unmistakable quality Professor Yun was taking about - INWARD CALM."[116] A more conservative estimate of Li Ching-Yun's age placed him at 197 years old, born in 1783.

Dr. Paavo Airola also gives a scientific reason why a low intake of protein is connected to a long life. "A high animal protein diet, is one of the main causes of senility and premature aging which has been recently stressed by two leading European biochemists and doctors - Professor Ph. Schwarz, of Frankfurt University, and Dr. Ralph Bircher of Zurich, Switzerland. They reported that the aging processes are triggered by a substance called *amyloid*, a by-product of protein metabolism, which is deposited in connective tissues and causes tissue and organ degeneration. Amyloid, the aging-producing substance, contains a large percentage of the amino acids tryptophan and tyrosine, which are plentiful in animal proteins.

"The connection between deposits of amyloid in the tissues and the degenerative diseases and aging processes in man has been known for a long time, but conveniently forgotten in this age of the high protein fad. Famous German pathologist, Dr. Rudolf Virchow, suggested as early as 1854 that amyloid deposits cause degenerative changes and premature aging. Amyloidosis was produced in experimental animals by feeding them high-protein diets."[117]

It is interesting if we go back to the Biblical Account of the Flood where God first allowed man to eat meat and also said his life span would be only 120 years, whereas before it was over 800 years old. On a strict vegetarian diet with fruit and vegetable based protein this amyloid problem is minimized, but with meat it is accentuated. During the Garden of Eden, 'the age of innocence,' was the time that man was living the strict raw vegan diet and he lived a long, long life, over 800 years. Afterwards during the age of man's 'heart contriving evil,' when he could eat meat, his life dropped to 120 years.

It should be stated that a vegetarian diet is an alkaline diet and all the longest lived populations had this alkaline diet. Most all the major nature oriented healing centers use an alkaline based diet to heal major illness. The human pH is 7.43 which is slightly on the alkaline side and sickness usually happens when the body chemistry is in an acid state. The Standard American Diet (meat eaters) is on the acid side of the pH scale.

In a book on: *How to Prolong Life: An Enquiry into the Cause of Old Age and Natural Death*, written over a hundred years ago by Dr. Charles Evans of England, there was a review of a study of centenarians in England in the

1800's. Dr. Evans said: "On reviewing nearly 2000 reported cases of persons who lived more than a century, we generally find some peculiarity of diet or habits to account for their alleged longevity; we find some were living amongst all the luxuries life could afford, others in the most abject poverty - begging their bread; some were samples of symmetry and physique, others cripples; some drank large quantities of water, others little; some were total abstainers form alcoholic drinks, others drunkards; some smoked tobacco, others did not; some lived entirely on vegetables, others to a great extent on animal foods; some led active lives, others sedentary; some worked with their brain, others with their hands; some ate only one meal a day, others four or five; some few ate large quantities of food, others a small amount; in fact, we notice great divergence both in habits and diet, but in those cases where we have been able to obtain a reliable account of the diet, we find one great cause which accounts for the majority of cases of longevity, *moderation in the quantity of food.*"

Obviously this study was done on people who lived before the modern age with all our toxins and poisons that we have today. But this is a basic principle in a healthy diet, to eat sparingly. This makes sense since less food means less wear and tear on the body.

In a medical journal, Dr. Jeremiah Stamler, a cardiologist was talking about lifestyles and demonstrating with statistics on death rate quotes, he noted that: "An additional comparison has recently become available, with data on mortality; for three groups of Californian Seventh Day Adventists (non-vegetarian, lacto-ovo-vegetarian and pure vegetarian) compared with the Californian general population. Seventh Day Adventists have lower mean serum cholesterol levels than Americans generally. For 47,000 Seventh Day Adventist men aged 35 and over, age-sex-standardized, mortality rates were 34% lower for non-vegetarians, 57% lower for the lacto-ovo-vegetarians and 77% lower for the pure vegetarians compared to the general population. Seventh Day Adventists differ from the general population in other respects as well, e.g. abstinence from both alcohol and tobacco." The results were evident that the strict dietary standards by the Adventists made them much healthier. The Adventist men had a heart attack mortality rate only 12 percent that of the average California male. Lung cancer was reduced 80 percent; uterine cancer in women was reduced 46 percent. In nearly every major disease, Adventist ranked well below the average in risk.[118] And they lived an average of ten years longer than the average California person.

"Scientific data suggest positive relationships between a vegetarian diet and reduced risk for several chronic degenerative diseases and conditions, including obesity, coronary artery disease, hypertension, diabetes mellitus, and some types of cancer." *Journal of the American Dietetic Association*[119] "Vegetarians often have lower mortality rates from several chronic degenerative diseases than do non-vegetarians." *British Medical Journal* [120]

A Dr. Edward Stiegbitz in his book, *The Second Forty Years*, points out that: "Superficially, the answer is simple; intrinsically, extremely complex.... **The quality of the cellular environment is the determining factor**, whether the cells be growing in vitro in a test-tube, in vivo, in the living and functioning organism." There was a study done with a chicken heart, in which the chicken heart was kept alive for many years by daily cleansing the heart by the fluid it was in, until one weekend a graduate student forgot to do the cleansing and it died.

One study showed that fasting (diet restriction) is the only consistently proven method of extending lifespan and this article hypothesizes that it is because it reduces the total amount of oxidative stress within an animal. Technically speaking: Oxygen destroys mitochondrial genomes which lack DNA repair mechanisms. Diet restriction can attenuate age associate mitochondrial enzymatic dysfunction.[121]

Fasting optimizes the body for maximum effectiveness, because fasting is cleansing and detoxifying the liver, the large intestine and many other organs and parts of the body on a fast. *Fasting also catabolizes dying, dead and disease cells, allowing a healthier body.*

The conclusion is simple, people who fast, have inner calm, and have moderation on a vegetarian diet will live longer and healthier.

2. Yoga Disciplines

Yoga has various disciplines that are beneficial for purification purposes. Hatha Yoga is not an exercise even though most people think of it that way. In a yoga posture, the body, breath, rhythm or flow, nerves, brain and mind are all involved. While this is going on it needs to be a flowing meditation with the body and mind. Thus the benefit of the *asana*, or posture is beyond just stretching. This is a purification not just of the physical body but also the personality, mind and emotions. The benefits have brought remission and healing to many people for their aliments. A few possible types of yoga are:

a. Rosary Yoga, Beads Yoga
Rosary Yoga (or Beads yoga) is a yoga devotion (bhakti yoga). The rosary is a meditation it involves meditating on the mysteries of Jesus life while praying Our Father's, Hail Mary's and Gloria's. There are five sets of beads on a rosary they all start with an Our Father then ten Hail Mary's and a Glory Be. The Rosary yoga can be done in standing postures or just in sitting postures. On the Our Father is a sitting posture usually a lotus or cross legged pose. The ten Hail Mary's are a decade and are ten related postures (10 stretching forward, or 10 twisting, or 10 inversions, or 10 stretching upwards, or 10 gut moves). The Glory Be's are sitting with the head bowed or forward. During each decade a different mystery is meditated upon, there are 20 mysteries,

four different rosary mysteries that can be said. It takes 25-30 minutes but sometimes just a decade or two is enough. Just saying the rosary as a meditation by itself can be very helpful in getting to sleep. Oftentimes it works for me and has worked for many others. Maybe doing a rosary yoga routine can be of benefit for those with sleep problems? For more information: www.jimtibbetts.com

b. Prana Christus Yoga

The term "prana" means human spirit and "Prana" with a capital P implies the Holy Spirit or part of it. All humans are body, soul and spirit. Healing can start with the human spirit and come through the human soul into the body, or it can come from the energy of the Holy Spirit through the human spirit or sometimes directly from the Holy Spirit, which is rare though. Prana Christus Yoga means the Spirit of Jesus yoga (*Christus* is a latin word for Christ) that involves praise and the spirit of healing. Getting into the spirit of praise and invoking the holy name of Jesus brings blessings and healing. Praise is a form of chanting which is often done in yoga, this is often found in bhakti yoga which can bring remission and healing.

c. Yoga Pilates

Pilates is an exercise routine that was developed by an American Joseph Pilates, which became very popular in the 50's, 60's 70's and still is popular today. About 50% of all Pilates moves are really yoga postures with movement put to them. Some yoga teachers do a combined class of yoga and Pilates which is very popular and could be therapeutically very beneficial. Pilates concentrates on the core for many moves and may appeal to some people over yoga or its movement activity could be more helpful then yoga for their sleep problems. A person would have to try it for a few months to see if it works for them.

d. Vegetus Yoga

Vegetus Yoga is a type of yoga that is nutritionally based in a plant-based diet for the purpose of purification.

This discipline of yoga involves those who are vegetarians, vegans and raw vegans. Yoga is a discipline of purification which has various types: Hatha, Raja, Prana, Bhakti, Jana, Karma, Mantra, Vegetus and other types of yoga. The Latin term *"vegetus"* means living or alive is often used for those who call themselves, "vegetarians". The Latin word, *vegetus* is the root for vegetarian. This is the type of food group (living foods) often used in the healing process of chronic diseases. All raw plant-based foods like vegetables and fruits are "living foods" before processing and are usually in their optimum nutritional state.

3. Increased Oxygen

High levels of oxygen are beneficial for the body, especially for degenerative diseases. Raw fruits and vegetables and juices have high levels of oxygen, cooked and processed foods have low levels of oxygen. All this cooking along with the smog and air pollution has reduced the amounts of oxygen we take in. Raw foods have the most oxygen. Dr. John Gainer in *Science News* wrote, "On a high-fat and high-protein diet, our oxygen supply is greatly reduced." He stated, "that even a moderate increase in blood-plasma protein can reduce oxygen levels of the blood by as much as 60 percent."[122]

A Bedroom Greenhouse - A second way to get more oxygen naturally is through a greenhouse. Have you ever walked through an enclosed greenhouse and taken a deep breath? Plants give off oxygen, which is noticeable whether the plants are in a greenhouse or your bedroom. If you put many big leafy plants in your bedroom and living room, they give off oxygen and clean the air in the room. This higher level of oxygen in the air increases the quality of oxygen you breathe into your body. This would help to build your immune system and fight degenerative diseases.

Juices and Smoothies - Another way to get more oxygen into the body is through drinking many freshly made juices. At the Gerson clinic, they emphasis 13- 8 oz. glasses of freshly made raw juice every day, one glass every hour. Of course, there are several reasons for this, one reason being that many nutrients and phytonutrients are entering the body through the juice. A second reason that is often overlooked is the amount of extra oxygen that is taken in. When juice is freshly made, many oxygen molecules end up being attached to the molecules in the juice. These are transported to the cells in the body. These added oxygen molecules in the cellular structure of the freshly made juice are incorporated into the body, raising the level of oxygen in the body naturally. This extra oxygen is an influence in helping the body to cure degenerative diseases.

4. Sunshine Needs

Sunshine influences the body in many ways that will be beneficial for the body and brain and thus for sleep too. In an abstract by the Vitamin D Council (2010),[3] they propose that vitamin D plays a role in mental illness based on the following five reasons:

1. Epidemiological evidence shows an association between reduced sun exposure and mental illness.
2. Mental illness is associated with low 25-hydroxyvitamin D [25(OH)D] levels.
3. Mental illness shows significant co morbidity with illnesses thought to be associated with vitamin D deficiency.
4. Theoretical models (*in vitro* or animal evidence) exist to explain how vitamin D deficiency may play a causative role in mental illness.
5. Studies indicate vitamin D improves mental illness.

Sunshine on the skin is an essential component of beauty and health. Denser bones, stronger muscles, richer blood, healthier nerves, and greater endurance are created by

---

[3] www.vitamindcouncil.org

regular exposure to sunshine. Understand that over-sunning, like over-eating, is harmful. Over-sunning causes free-radical collagen damage to the skin.[123]

Twenty minutes a day would be fine; half an hour or more and may promote sunburn, depending on the person's skin type. Sunshine several times a week would be very helpful. For otherwise healthy persons, the FNB reports adequate intake (AI) for vitamin D is 200, 400, or 600 IU a day, depending on your age. But Dr. Robert Heaney, et al, writing in the *American Journal of Clinical Nutrition* in 2003 said: "The recommendations of the Food and Nutrition Board with respect to oral vitamin D input fall into a curious zone between irrelevance and inadequacy. For those persons with extensive solar exposure, the recommended inputs add little to their usual daily production, and for those with no exposure, the recommended doses are insufficient to ensure desired 25(OH)D concentration."[124] (*New Engl Jour Med*)

Michael Holick's, MD, PhD (in 1995), demonstration "that a brief dose of noontime summer sun is comparable to taking between 10,000–25,000 IU of vitamin D. Four earlier papers all found similar amounts of natural vitamin D production. Adam *et al,* found that up to 50,000 IU of vitamin D was released into the circulation of Caucasians after 30 minutes of noontime summer sun."[125] "A minimum of 5,000 IU of vitamin D a day is needed (from all sources, diet, sun and supplements) as recognized by various studies."[126]

Dr. Michael Holick (Boston University, an expert on sunlight) now believes "that a full body minimal erythemal dose of summer sunlight at noontime produces 20,000 IU of vitamin D. The high amount of natural human production of vitamin D is the single most important fact every physician should know about vitamin D because it has such profound implications for the natural human condition. Furthermore, there has never been a reported case of vitamin D intoxication due to excessive sun-exposure such as lifeguards, sun-worshippers, etc. The reason is that once the skin makes enough vitamin D, the sun destroys the excess. Some rather technical benefits in other studies can be cited, but the end result is that yes, there is a connection between brain health and having enough sunlight."[127]

IX. Nutrition After the Fast

The best type of nutrition to move into after the fast is a plant-based diet and the highest type of plant-based diet is the category of raw vegan or Living Foods.

1. Fasting improves absorption

Fasting is important to improve nutrient absorption. Dr. Shelton, a leading fasting expert this century points out that, "fasting has been shown to be beneficial in certain deficiency states (scurvy, beriberi, rickets, iron deficiency). He further states that fasting does not produce vitamin deficiency the way unbalanced diets do and claims that dietary imbalance can lead to death much quicker than complete fasting. He theorizes that fasting improves deficiency states by increasing the ability of tissues to absorb and utilize nutrients.[128] Therefore fasting increases the tissues ability to absorb nutrients; such as vitamins and minerals and other important food nutrients.

Diet is also very important. In one vegetarian study; 50,000 Seventh Day Adventist in California were compared with those for average Californians. The results were evident that the strict dietary standards by the Adventist made them much healthier. The Adventist men had a heart attack mortality rate only 12 percent that of the average California male. Lung cancer was reduced 80 percent; Uterine cancer in women was reduced 46 percent. In nearly every major disease, Adventist ranked well below the average in risk.[129] In addition they lived an average of ten years longer than the average California person.

It is often best to start out with the basics. There are five categories of foods that need to be avoided and are often called the Five Whites.

- First - refined sugar, which is actually a drug.
- Second is dairy that is pasteurized (heating to 160 degrees or higher).
- Third is salt, which is needed in the body in a natural organic form, not the inorganic table salt usually sold. (Most vegetables like celery contain salt in its organic form.)
- Fourth is white flour which has all the good substances (bran and germ) taken out during processing.
- Fifth would be animal products, especially the white fat in meat.
- The five whites all have three things in common:
   1. No fiber in any of these products;
   2. Cooking and processing gives them little if any nutrients;
   3. They become toxic and drug- like in their effects.

The diet of an animal usually relates to its physiological structure. There are meat eating animals and non-meat eating or vegetarian (grass and leaf) eating animals. And there are a few animals like the apes that are fruit and nut eating animals. Apes are the strongest animals on earth for their size. A silver-back gorilla has 30 times the strength and only 3 times the size of man. These gorillas "eat nothing but fruit and bamboo leaves and can turn your car over if they wanted to."[130]

The term 'vegetarian' does not mean 'vegetable eater' but it stems from the Latin *vegetus,* which means 'whole, sound, fresh, and lively,' or 'to enliven'. Most vegetarians believe that plant foods are life giving, alive and bring health. The word 'diet' comes from the Greek word *dieta*, which means 'way of life'. A diet needs to be a lifestyle in order to be effective.

Plant-based diets can be divided into three general categories: vegetarian, vegan and raw vegan. The vegetarians sometimes add milk or cheese or eggs (lacto-ovo-vegetarians or even fish); yet vegans have not animals products. Most of the time people start out as a vegetarian, and then move to being a vegan and then to raw vegan, which is the highest or purest form of eating. Many if not most grains are problematic and cooking destroys a lot of the nutrients in foods.

For a Raw Vegan or Living Foods Diet these four categories are usually considered base foods and grains are very limited in use:
1. Vegetables green and leafy vegetables, etc.)
2. Legumes (beans and peas of all sorts)
3. Fruits (apples, oranges, plums, etc.)
4. Nuts and Seeds (almonds, walnuts, peanuts, etc.)
5. Grains (rice, barley, millet, wheat, bulgur, etc.) - used in a limited way.

Raw Living foods are Superior to Cooked foods.
Fresh, raw living foods contain all the nutrients necessary for good health, growth, maintenance and repair. Living foods avoid the stimulant highs and depressant lows (sugar, coffee, tea, coke, rich foods, overeating, alcohol, etc.).

Living foods are easier to prepare and digest.
Living foods are much easier to clean up after.
Living foods help the body to achieve a normal weight.
Living foods restore the natural *appestat* (appetite control).
Living foods do not cause or support degenerative diseases.
Living foods help a person feel better and have more energy.
Living foods give the highest possible nutrient count
        per calorie.
Living foods allow a person to spend less time sleeping.
Living foods eliminate bad breath, body odor and halitosis.
Living foods cost less when it becomes a lifestyle.

Cooking, baking roasting, broiling, boiling and steaming destroy from 30% to 90% of the nutrition in the food, resulting in a nutrient-deficient diet, the main cause of degenerative diseases. 100% of the enzymes are destroyed in cooking. Minerals are lost when cooking, liquids (broth) are poured out.

Cooked foods become so devitalized they take more energy than they give and are difficult to digest.

Cooked foods shorten our life span.

Cooked foods cause far more build-up of toxins, a factor suppressing the immune system and making the body more susceptible to disease of all kinds.

Cooked foods encourage over eating, resulting in weight gain. Since they are nutrient-deficient, they leave the system still hungering for and craving food.

Cooked foods falsely satisfy the taste and appetite but cause abnormal cravings for sugar foods (candy, cakes, pies, ice creams, cookies, etc.) Heavy meats, richly seasoned starches, such as breads with spreads, deep fat-fried potato and corn chips, French fries, spicy, rich grain and legume dishes also cause abnormal cravings. After such a meal, the coffee drinker craves coffee, which over-stimulates the pancreas to produce more enzymes to digest all that heavy food.[131]

Living Foods are raw, generally if not mostly uncooked. The Supermarket is mostly a Foods Funeral Home, with dead foods lying in state! On grocery shelves there sit more than 5,000 items processed from whole natural foods into empty edibles. Some 65% of the American adult and 25% of children under 17 now live with chronic disease and medication.

Heat is one of the main destroyers of nutrients in your food. Enzymatic destruction begins at 116 degrees, vitamins lose potency at 130 degrees, and proteins become denatured above 161 degrees, Fahrenheit. Dehydration of foods under 116 degrees preserves the nutrients.[132]

In the US there is the American Dietetic Association which most nutritionists belong too, it states: "Studies indicate that vegetarians often have lower morbidity and mortality rates . . . Not only is mortality from coronary artery disease lower in vegetarians than in non vegetarians, but vegetarian diets have also been successful in arresting coronary artery disease. Scientific data suggest positive relationships between a vegetarian diet and reduced risk for... obesity, coronary artery disease, hypertension, diabetes mellitus, and some types of cancer."

American Dietetic Association
Position Paper on Vegetarian Diets

A lot of the healing clinics and alternative healing centers use vegetarian diet therapy to help heal with Raw Living Foods Diets are the main plant-based diets used in diet therapy. Even though there are different versions of raw vegan diets, they are all pretty similar since they use mostly, if not totally, raw living foods.

What kinds of things can Diet Therapy heal? Just about everything. The Gerson diet at one hospital has for over twenty years specialized in the treatment of:

- Cancer; Melanoma; Multiple Myeloma; Hodgkins disease; Heart disease; Diabetes; Hypertension; Lupus; Arthritis; Alzheimer's; Candida; Crohn's Disease; Chronic Fatigue Syndrome; Migraine headaches; Liver disease; Kidney disease; Thyroid disease; Allergies and other degenerative diseases.
- And this is just one hospital that uses raw living foods, juicing and supplements in diet therapy.

A German raw fooder, Dr. Johann Georg Schnitzer has helped many people learn to eat living foods and did a major study showing its benefits. Following are a few of the benefits in his monumental study. The study involved 4702 people and their 2700 children who were questioned on how they had become healthier, more efficient and content. The

Schnitzer-Report is 548 pages with tables, graphs and statistical analysis by the Institute for Demoscopy in Germany, about people following the Schnitzer-Nutritional recommendations.

A few of the findings without mentioned all the statistics for each are:
- constipation fewer colds,
- influenza
- spared the German measles;
- didn't get the chicken pox
- didn't get the measles;
- no children's diseases at all
- Psychological disposition of these children also improved.
- less tooth decay;
- an improvement with their gum problems;
- On the living foods diet, among the men: 92.7% felt more productive than before the change and 71.2% are tired less often.
- Among the women, they became more energetic after the change-over: 91.7% indicated greater productivity; 76.6% were tired less often; 17.8% never felt tired again.

One of the greatest therapies is to have these degenerative diseases is to enter the Green Zone. On the Living Foods diet you eat a lot of produce, especially greens and after a while a person desires greens, and salads and vegetables. For degenerative disease, a person needs to enter into and stay in the, Green Zone!

It's all about purification, not just purification of the body, but purification of the soul which includes mind, emotions and will. Some people have a mindset that needs to be purified or educated to think correctly or purely. Gluttony is the eating of too much food or drink, or eating too much of the wrong type of food or drink. As St. Thomas Aquinas (d.

1274) states, 'There are seven capital sins or vices: pride, covetousness, gluttony, lust, envy, anger and sloth. They are disordered inclinations.'[133]   Gluttony is a major sin/vice in the United States and in most developed countries.

Food and fasting are taught as part of the way of those who follow God's Holy Word in the Bible. This principle is often referred to as Kosher. Kosher means 'pure,' or is a reference to pure food, which is helpful in the process of purification. Purity is one of the main concepts in the bible. We are meant to be pure and holy, which go hand and hand, because we have a physical body, with a soul and human spirit. We do purification or penance to purify our physical body and soul, to keep it whole and holy!

The purest type of kosher is a plant-based diet. These are the principles of the bible and of Christ Jesus and not the principles of the world. The principles of the world include all the many scientists, medical doctors and diet gurus writings books, articles, and some who are on television.

For more detailed information on plant-based diets and Biblical Nutrition see the author's other books. The first principle of the bible on food is found in Genesis 1:29. "God said, 'See, I give you all the seed-bearing plants that are upon the whole earth, and all the trees with seed-bearing fruit; this shall be your food.'" Man's original diet was a raw vegan diet, which included no animal products and no cooking. Most of the degenerative diseases are influenced by or caused by animal products and cooking. Today in the area of nutrition, "My people are being destroyed from lack of knowledge." Hos 4:6

2. The Alleluia Nutrition Therapy

The Alleluia diet is founded by Jim Tibbetts, STL, MBA (a Catholic theologian) and Anne Marie Tibbetts, MS, RD (registered dietitian with over 24 years of experience). The Alleluia diet goes along with the Alleluia Nutrition

Therapy (Six Sigma Nutrition Therapy for the secular environment)! It hopes that people can become whole and get healed in their body, soul and spirit, and then can shout with joy, "Alleluia!" A Lifestyle approach: body, soul, spirit.

One of the greatest therapies for ill health is to first enter the Green Zone then later to enter the Blue Zone of Fasting. Several long fasts are needed to cure these major degenerative diseases. A person needs to enter into the rainbow of plant-based foods and their colors, especially green in their nutritional therapy. To help achieve and remain in the Alleluia Nutrition therapy recommends at least two or three of these every day:
- o a green smoothie
- o green or other colors superfoods
- o a shot of wheat or barley grass or other green
- o a glass or several glasses of green juice
- o a large salad with Kale and/or other greens
❖ Several glasses of green juice, Super Greens every day, a large salad with greens daily, green smoothies, juices and powders daily, green superfoods, low-fat raw vegan and emphasizing fruits.

Green smoothies contain green vegetables and fruits. There are many variations. The benefit of green smoothies to sleep disorder patients is not just in the extremely healthy mixture just mentioned above, but that it gives a place to add supplements in a tasty way.

The term 80/20 Raw is internationally accepted to mean, 80% raw and 20% cooked in a raw vegan diet. It is the "80/20 raw vegan threshold" that is the doorway to healing most degenerative diseases, as evidence suggests from various health professionals and case studies. Yet a 95% to a 100% raw vegan diet is the ideal and should be sought after. The Alleluia diet (Six Sigma diet) emphasizes a nutrition therapy approach as follows:

- A 100%/95% Live-Food diet is the ideal. People with major degenerative diseases should try to reach 100% raw foods the first year.
- Optional, an 85/15% raw vegan diet, usually one meal is a large salad; this is a 100% vegan, 85% raw plant-based foods, which has less than 15% cooked foods.
- Six 8 oz. glasses of freshly-juiced carrot juice daily; freshly-juiced apple or cucumber juice or other veggie juice may replace part of the carrot juice
- Six teaspoons of a green powder like barley grass powder (taken 2 to 3 times) a day
- A green or rainbow colored smoothie every day
- Breakfast should be juice, a smoothie, some fruit, or a light meal (fermented foods could be at this meal)
- Lunch and Dinner consists of two large raw vegan meals (one is a large salad and some fermented foods)
- Exercises like yoga, Pilates or walking at least ½ hour a day to help digestion; include some sunshine, fresh air and prayer daily.
- Finally, a weekly or bi-monthly meeting or conversation with a health professional, counselor or health coach is advised to work through the issues, both past and present.

So in summary:
1. Two to three raw vegan meals; lunch and dinner one is a large salad, some fermented food or drink
2. Six 8oz glasses of freshly juiced carrot and/or apple, cucumber and/or fresh juice (not pasteurized)
3. Three to Six teaspoons of a barley grass or wheat grass or a mixture of green grasses as a powder, a day."

After getting going on the nutrition protocol for a couple of weeks, just described, a long fast should be undertaken. A 14 to28 day juice fast, or a water fast under supervision should be taken. This first fast will probably not cure the disease but it will start the process of eliminating poisons, detoxifying other things and starting to reset the biochemistry back to its normal status. Over the course of a year, three long fast will probably be needed. The lengths will differ but these could help bring a complete remission of the disease along with the above protocol.

(The above is a basic outline of the diet and fasting which goes along with the other things mentioned in this book, such as supplements.)

3. Lifestyle Medicine LFP Methodology

The approach used here is primarily Evidence-Based Nutrition, but also taken into account are the journal studies and experience from Evidence-Based Medicine, using a Lifestyle Medicine LFP approach. Lifestyle Medicine is an approach to medicine which is international with independent branches around the world. Yet the definition of Lifestyle Medicine in various countries and organization differs, and many do not emphasis a plant-based lifestyle. (Lifestyle Medicine LFP was designed specifically for this series on degenerative disease. LFP means L for Live-Foods or Living Plant-based Nutrition; F for fasting (water or juice fasting) or detoxification methods; and P for prayer and meditation methods.)

This book will describe the three pillars (LFP) as a methodology of curing, putting into remission and helping people with sleep disorders. The major focus is primarily a nutritional (what goes in) and fasting or detox (what comes out) approach. The three main categories in Lifestyle Medicine LFP are:

By the Person on himself – primary focus
1. Live-Foods or Living Plant-based Nutrition
    and supplementation
    and sunshine, oxygen and rest
    (These are what goes into the body)

2. Fasting: Juice and/or Water or Detox methods
    and curative exercises

and detoxification methods (& Ayruvedic)
(These are what detoxes, out of the body)

3. Prayer and meditation,
      and counseling or coaching
      and Ayruvedic medicine personality differences
      (These involve in/out in the soul or spirit)

There is a secondary approach by a Medical Doctor or Expert – the secondary focus is an alternative medical approach and to be used only when necessary and involves:
4. Pharmaceutical drugs
5. Surgery and other Allopathic approaches

Vegetarianism dates back thousands of years. During biblical times, the emphasis on Live-Foods or raw foods was found in a few groups such as the Jewish Essenes. In biblical times, everything was organic, natural, ripe, raw and fresh! The standard vegetarian diet today includes a lot of processed foods (healthy junk foods) and the quality varies widely. The Live-food, plant based diet approach is a whole new evolution in the plant-based field. Yet the truth is Live-Foods and fasting are counter-cultural.

Colin Campbell, PhD, professor emeritus of Cornell University, was part of the famous Women's Health Study and once asked the lead doctor of the study why they didn't show the real facts that the use of the plant-based diet orientation was a success in this study. This professor replied, "Because that's not what the public wants to hear!"[134] Reformers and new thinkers often times have a hard time promoting their discoveries. Max Gerson, MD, a medical doctor in the 40's and 50's, published 55 scientific works during his fifty years of practice and created the Gerson diet. He became famous for curing cancer and in his cancer book he states, "The history of medicine reveals that reformers who bring new ideas into the general thinking and practice of physicians have a difficult time."

X. Fasting Scripture and Spirituality

"On a fast day...you shall read the words of the Lord."
Jeremiah 36.6

The Bible is the greatest book on fasting. Biblical references to the word "fasting," the reference to a partial fast, abstinence, or to the act of fasting, in Scripture, is given here. As you can see there is much more to fasting then just scientific approach and physiological benefits outlined in this book.

The Torah: Gn 3:3, God gave the first commandment which involved not eating. Gen 18.8, the angels follow the customs of men while on earth; Gen 24.33, Abraham's servant sent to choose a wife for Isaac; Exod 34.28, Moses' first forty-day fast on Mt. Sinai; Lev 16.29,31, The Day of Atonement; Lev 23.6, The Passover Abstinence; Lev 23.14, The first sheaf offering abstinence; Lev 23.27,32, the Day of Atonement; Num 6.1-4, the Nazirite vow; Num 29.7, the Day of Atonement; Deut 9.9,18, Moses' forty-day fast, twice;

The Historical Books: Jg 13.4, the Nazirite vow for Samson; Jg 20.26, the Israelites fasted and defeated the Benjamites; 1 Sam 1.7,8, Hannah refused to eat during the pilgrimage; 1 Sam 7.6, the Israelites fasted and defeated the Philistines; 1 Sam 14.24, Saul's oath to fast during battle; 1 Sam 20.34, Jonathan grieved at Saul's resolve to kill David; 1 Sam 28.20, Saul's despair at Samuel's message; 1 Sam 30.12; David feeds the Egyptian who had no nourishment for three days; 1 Sam 31.13, the seven day fast after Saul's burial; 2 Sam 1.12, David and his men mourning and fasting seven days at Saul's death; 2 Sam 3.35, David refused to eat before sunset at Abner's death; 2 Sam 11.11, Uriah's personal discipline in the time of war; 2 Sam 12.16,21.22, David's grief and repentance before Bathsheba's child's death; 1 Kg 13.8,16, the prophet who prophesied against the altar; 1 Kg 17.6, Elijah's restricted diet; 1 Kg 17.14-16,

Elijah and the widow and son's bread and water fast; 1 Kg 19.8, Elijah's forty day waling fast to Mt. Horeb; 1 Kg 21.4, King Ahab laying down on his bed would not eat; 1 Kg 21.9,12, Ahab's wife proclaimed a fast for Ahab; 1 Kg 21.27, Ahab's repentance and fasting saved his life; 1 Chr 10.12, the Jabeshgilead warriors recovered Saul's dead body and fasted seven days; 2 Chr 20.3, Jehoshaphat proclaimed a fast for all Judah and obtained victory in battle; Ezra 8.21,23, Ezra proclaimed a fast for their safe journey which was granted; Ezra 9.3,4, Ezra's denunciation of mixed marriages remains motionless; Ezra 10.6, Ezra's mourning the betrayal by the exiles; Neh 1.4, Nehemiah's prayer and fasting for Jerusalem; Neh 9.1, Ezra's reading from the Torah proclaiming fasting; Tb 12.8, Tobit delivered Sarah through Raphael's instructions; Judith 8.6, Judith fasted all the days of her widowhood; Est 4.3, the Jews fasting and weeping their sentence of destruction, Est 4.16, Esther's proclamation of the three day total fast; Est 9.31, Esther's fast is successful to save the Jewish race; 1 Mac 3.17, Judas and his army, weak from fasting, defeated the Gentiles by Heaven's strength; 1 Mac 3.47, Judas and the Israelite again defeated a larger army of Gentiles through prayer and fasting; 2 Mac 13.12, Judas and his men ward off the Syrians after three days of prayers, prostrations and fasting.

The Wisdom Books: Job 1.20-2.13, Job's morning ritual silently sitting on the ground; Job 33.20, Elihu's speech and appetite; Ps 35.13, David intercedes with prayer and fasting; Ps 42.1.3, the thirsting soul's food is tears; Ps 69.11, David's lament humbled himself with fasting; Ps 102.4, a loss of appetite during distress; Ps 107.18, food became repugnant during distress; the cause of David's physical weakness; Sir 34.26, true worship with fasting.

The Prophetic Books: Is 58, the kind of fasting which pleases God; Jer 14.12, that which is unacceptable to God; Jer 36.6, 9, Baruch reading Jeremiah's scroll on a fast day; Dan 1.12-16, Daniel and his companions refuse the king's food; Dan 6.18, Darius when Daniel was in the lions' den;

Dan 9.3, Daniel praying for Jerusalem; Dan 10.2,3, Daniel's three weeks' partial fast,; Joel 1.14, in view of the Day of the Lord,: Joel 2.12, when returning to God with all the heart; Joel 2.15, proclaimed by blowing a trumpet in Zion; Jonah 3.5-9, Jonah proclaimed by the people and the king of Nineveh; Zech 7.3-5, with mourning in the fifth and seventh months; Zech 8.19, kept in the fourth (April), fifth (May), seventh (July) and tenth (October) months.

The Four Gospels: Matt 4.2, the forty day fast of Jesus; Matt 6.16-18, not to be practiced as the hypocrites do; Mat 9.14,15, by the Pharisees and John's disciples; Matt 9.15, by the guests when the bridegroom has departed; Matt 11.18, the character of John the Baptist; Matt 15.32 the four thousand were hungry before our Lord fed them; Matt 17.21, this kind can only come forth by it; Mk 2.18, by John's disciples and the Pharisees; Mk 2.19,20, by the guests when the bridegroom has departed; Mk 8.3 the hungry four thousand fed by Jesus; Mk 9.29, only cast out by it; Lk 2.37, by Anna worshiping in the temple; Lk 4.2 the forty day fast of Jesus; Lk 5.33, by John's disciples and the Pharisees; Lk 5.34,35, by the guests when the bridegroom has departed; Lk 7.33, the character of John the Baptist; Lk 18.12, by the Pharisee, twice a week.

The Acts and Letters: Acts 9.9, Saul after his encounter with Christ; Acts 10.30; by Cornelius when an angel appeared to him; Acts 13.2,3, by prophets and teachers in Antioch; Acts 14.23, at the appointment of elders in the churches; Acts 23.12-21, by Jews under an oath to kill Paul; Acts 27.9, allusion to the annual Day of Atonement; Acts 27.21,33, by those with Paul before the shipwreck; Rom 14.21, abstaining for the sake of a weaker brother; 1 Cor 7.5, in the marriage relationship; 1 Cor 8.13, abstaining for the sake of a weaker brother; 2 Cor 11.27, in the list of Paul's sufferings; 1 Tim 4.3, false teachers commanding abstinence.

"In each of these churches they appointed elders, and with prayer and fasting they commended them to the Lord in whom they had come to believe." Acts 14:23

"Someone asked him, 'Lord, will only a few people be saved?' He answered them, 'Strive to enter through the narrow gate, for many, I tell you will attempt to enter but will not be strong enough.'" Lk 13:22-30

"But now, now - it is Yahweh who speaks - come back to me with all your heart, fasting, weeping and mourning." Joel 2:1

If Moses, who beheld God, (on Sinai) and St. Paul, the divine apostle (Act 9:9) fasted, so must we. If the Ninevites fasted (Jonah 3:5), and this included all their children plus their 'senior' citizens, so we must. If the Church Fathers and the Saints fasted, and expected others to fast, so must we. Finally, if Jesus Himself fasted and was hungry (Lk 4:2), who are we to introduce a 'new improved and fast-free' spirituality?

From scriptures to the early Church Fathers fasting is part of the Christian way of life. Clement of Alexandria (d. 202), making use of scripture and philosophy, recommends frugality and temperance to free oneself from matter.[135] For Origen, fasting is an experience of freedom, not an obligation in view of Pythagorean metapsychosis.[136] For Ambrose and Gregory of Nyssa, mortification of the flesh puts man in communion with Christ who raises him from human to a divine existence.[137] For Basil, fasting guarantees peace in the world and in families, because it frees people from egoism.[138] And for Ambrose, it is the angelic life that leads us back to Paradise, where 'sin entered through food'; 'those who do not believe in the afterlife indulge in food and drink.'"[139]

"Monasticism carried the ascesis of fasting to incredible heights. Anthony ate bread, water and salt.[140] Pachomius fasted, but did not want his monks to lack food.[141] For Jerome, the monk must always remain a little hungry: 'If you wish to be perfect, it is better to fatten the soul than the body.'[142] Basil and Cassian recommended moderation, each one adapting the fast to his own situation.[143] St. Benedict's (d. 547) *Rule* recommends us to 'love fasting' with discretion.[144] While the monastic East explored the personal aspect, the Western communities looked to the social value. Leo the Great, who dedicated 30 treatises to fasting, said: 'the abstinence of him who fasts becomes the nourishment of the poor.'"[145]

From the time of the Early Church Fathers to the present time fasting has been emphasized in religious orders. The religious orders in the Church have all emphasized fasting to some degree. Some religious individuals and some canonized Saints have emphasized longer fasts, seven days and longer as a religious practice. St. Francis of Assisi and St. Francis of Paola are two saints that have emphasized longer fasts for their order and practiced longer fasts personally. St. Francis of Assisi fasted for 40 days numerous times and in his rule encouraged his Friars to fast. "All the friars without exception must fast from the feast of All Saints until Christmas, and from Epiphany, when our Lord began his fast, until Easter. The friars are not bound by the Rule to fast at other times, except on Friday."[146] And St. Francis of Paola also emphasized fasting in his rule.[147]

Spiritual/Psychological/Physical Benefits of Fasting

"Yet, when they were sick, I put sackcloth on, I humbled my soul with fasting." Ps 35:13

The number one question that people have asked me about a long fast is, "Why do you go on a long fast?" or "What is the benefit of a long fast?" The answer is three fold as follows:

Fasting benefits us on three levels: body, soul and spirit. First it benefits us in our human spirit in which it humbles the soul, allowing the human spirit to flourish and deepen. At times of a long fast the human spirit is able to flourish and open up to God, deepening its awareness of the Trinity and of God's Creation. It also opens us up to God's perfect Will for our lives, for the path that is best for us to take, for things we should be doing or avoiding, for future activities that we need to prepare for. Our prayer life is able to deepen in ways it hasn't before, insights and inspirations about our prayer life, relationship with others and with God deepen and move forward in a positive maturing direction. Our human spirit is purified of roots from the soul that need purification or other needed purification in the human spirit, so that our spirit might be purified and pure before God. There are many ways in our human spirit that matures and grows through a long fast these are a few.

The second benefit of fasting is in the human soul (the psyche) which consists of the mind, emotions or will (or in psychological terms the intelligence, affections and motivational components of our being). As scripture notes, the soul is humbled. The soul enters into a state of purification or lessening of vices connected to the mind, emotions and will. Without a stomach full of food or digestive system working hard we are able to think clearer and feel more effectively and be motivated in a stronger fashion. Our mind and emotions have clarity of thought to ponder and meditate more deeply on things in the temporal world that concern us. Our soul is able to let go of vices and problems (like addictions) and the soul matures to deal with these more effectively, both during and after coming off, the fast. There are many ways in our human soul that matures and grows through a long fast these are a few.

The third benefit of fasting is in the human body. The body is purified and body is allowed to restructure back to its perfect state of design or normality. It is common knowledge that there are certain health indicators such as blood pressure, or pH levels. These simple outer health indicators are biochemically or physiologically controlled and long fasts, such as a seven day fast, help to normalize these. Sometimes it takes several weeks on a fast or several long fasts but slowly the body moves back to it normal state of healthy design. This also happens on a cellular level biochemically. The imperfections or abnormalities on a cellular level start to normalize themselves. A second major thing fasting does (on a long fast) is that it catabolizes the dead, diseased and dying cells in the body and flushes them out. This is called internal house-cleaning. The adipose tissue (fat tissue) is the first to be cleansed and flushed out but then on a longer fast it goes much deeper into the tissues and cleanses these of diseases and other cellular abnormalities that are catabolized (cellular anabolism) and flushed out of the body. There are many ways in our human body is purified through a long fast these are a few; the first chapters in this book covers some of the other benefits to the body, as well as the section on therapeutic fasting.

The human body is integrated in with the human psyche which is integrated in with the human spirit, all three work together harmoniously. The roots of vice and illness can grow from the body to the soul and then influence the human spirit; or it can grow from the soul to the body and then influence the spirit; or it can start as sin in the spirit and then grow into the soul and this would eventually grow into the body. Fasting is a primary way to purify all three areas of our being: body, soul and spirit.

"But now, now - it is Yahweh who speaks - come back to me **with all your heart**, fasting, weeping, mourning." Joel 2:12

People today need to be "given instruction in the Way of the Lord." (Acts 18:25) Hopefully this book has helped to fulfill this command in the area of fasting.

XI. - Appendix

A. Bio - James C. Tibbetts

Jim Tibbetts has an MBA (2009); an STL (1995) in Marian Studies (International Marian Research Institute, Univ. Dayton, Ohio) and an MA (1983) in theology (Univ. Steubenville, Ohio). He is a member of Secular Franciscan Order, the K of C and the American Mariological Society. James as a businessman ran various businesses and has worked with the mentally handicapped. As a theologian he has given talks at national conferences, society meetings and given retreats on; Spirituality, Marian topics; on plant-based diets, fasting, healing and Christian meditation. He has been into a plant-based diet and seven day juice fasting since late 1970's and has done over 40 long juice fasts.

Jim produced several DVD's on spiritual topics and mime. From 1978 to 2003, Jim was a professional mime; solo, duet and was a founding member (1991 to 2001) of the group "Christsong" which performed around the U.S., twice-toured England and appeared on television shows. "Tibbetts has studied his art under technique-oriented Marcel Marceau and personality-oriented Tony Montanaro. The result has been a critically acclaimed combination of the two." (*Arts & Entertainment*, Evening Express, Portland, ME.)

Jim developed and leads the Rosary Yoga (and Pilates) with groups, a posture for each bead and he promotes Christian Yoga. He has written journal and popular articles and has written over 20 books including:

1. Juice Fasting Simplified, a Practical Approach
2. A Diary on Juice Fasting
3. Living Green with Juices, Smoothies and Salads with Anne Marie Tibbetts, MS, RD
4. Starving Cancer to Death, Nutritional Integrative Cancer Therapies, with Joseph Spaziani, MD

5. Starving into Remission: Alzheimer's, Parkinson's
    and Multiple Sclerosis - Nutritional Therapies
    with Anne Marie Tibbetts, MS, RD
6. The Bioethics of Drug Intervention
7. Superior Health for Astronauts as Raw Vegans
    A Nutrition Novel
8. Christian Meditation, the Jesus Prayer and Praise
9. Jesus and Mary were Kosher Vegetarian, the Evidence
    from the Bible, the Early Church and Nutrition (2014)
10. Biblical Nutrition and Fasting (2008)
11. Biblical Nutrition; Forty Days of Meditations (2004)
12. Biblical Nutrition the Kosher Vegetarianism
    of Jesus and Judaism (2003)
13. Biblical Fasting (1998)
14. A Biblical Ballad of Mary Mother of Jesus
15. Biblical Titles of the Virgin Mary - 30 Day Meditation
16. Mary the Kosher Vegetarian, Impacting Climate Change
17. Mary the Ark of the Covenant with Fr. Bill McCarthy
18. Guadalupe the Tilma's Conquest - a historical novel
19. Q&A about Vegetarians and Health

Jim Tibbetts
P.O. Box 2533
Glenville, NY 12325
www.jimtibbetts.com

Notice:

If this book is a significant help to your health or
illness or degenerative disease, or even beneficial or a
conversion or faith walk, please let us know. Myself and my
associates are collecting testimonials and case studies for
future works and possible a book. We are always interested
when this book helps you in you're: body, soul or spirit.
Drop us a letter. I do not always reply to email, but I always
reply to a snail mail, drop me a letter. Thank you and God
bless.   Sincerely in Christ
         Jim Tibbetts

B. Endnotes

[1] Levin, Buck, Ph.D., R.D., Environmental Nutrition: Understanding the Link between Environment, Food Quality, and Disease, Vashon Island, Washington, HingePin Integrative Learning Materials, 1999): p. 179, citing: Murphy R. and Harvey C. (1985). Residues and metabolites of selected persistent halogenated hydrocarbons in blood from a general population survey. *Environ Health Perspect* 60:115-120.

[2] Levin, Buck, Environmental Nutrition…, p. 179, citing: Lordo RA, Dinh KT, and Schwemberger JG. (1996). Semivolatile organic compounds in adipose tissue: estimated averages for the US population and selected subpopulations. *Am J Pub Heal* 86(9):1253-1259.

[3] Levin, Buck, Environmental Nutrition, p. 215, citing: Stehr-Green PA. (1989). Demographic and seasonal influences on human serum pesticide residue levels. J *Toxicol Environ Heal* 27(4):405-421.

[4] Levin, Buck, Environmental Nutrition, p. 181, citing: Henriksen GL, Ketchum NS, Michalek JE it al. (1997). Serum dioxin and diabetes mellitus in veterans of Operation Ranch Hand. *Epidem* 8(3):252-258.

[5] Levin, Buck, Environmental Nutrition, p. 181, citing: Hill RH Jr, Ashley DL, Head Sl et al. (1995). P-dichlorobenzene exposure among 1,000 adults in the United States. *Arch Environ Health* 50(4):277-280.

[6] Levin, Buck, Environmental Nutrition, p. 181, citing: Hammand TA, Sexton M, and Langenberg P. (1996). Relationship between blood lead and dietary iron intake in preschool children. *Ann Epidemiol* 6(1):30-33. Also: Kim R, Landrigan c, Mossmann P et al. (1997). Age and secular trends in bone lead levels in middle-aged and elderly men: three-year longitudinal follow-up in the Normative Aging Study. *Am J Epidemiol* 146(7):586-591.

[7] Levin, Buck, Environmental Nutrition, p. 181, citing: Yamamura Y, Yoshinaga Y, Arai F et al. (1994). Background levels of total mercury concentrations in blood and urine. *Sangyo Igaku* 36(2):66-69.

[8] Levin, Buck, Environmental Nutrition, p. 181, citing: Chia SE, chan OY, Sam CT et al. (1994). Blood cadmium levels in nonoccupationally exposed adult subjects in Singapore. *Sci Total Environ* 145(1-2): 119-123.

[9] Levin, Buck, Environmental Nutrition, p. 181, citing: Wolff MS, Anderson HA, and selikoff IJ. (1982). Human tissue burdens of halogenated aromatic chemicals in Michigan. *JAMA* 247(15):2112-2116.

[10] Levin, Buck, Environmental Nutrition, p. 181, citing: Hill RH Jr, Head SL, Baker S et al. (1995). Pesticide residues in urine of adults living in the United States: reference range concentrations. *Environ Res* 71(2): 99-108.

[11] Levin, Buck, Environmental Nutrition, p. 215, citing: Guengerich FP and Shimada T, *op. cit.*

[12] Levin, Buck, Environmental Nutrition, p. 215, citing: Nakajima T and Wang RS. (1994). Induction of cytochrome P450 by toluene. Int J Biochem 26(12):133301340.

[13] Levin, Buck, Environmental Nutrition, p. 215, citing: Ungv-rg G. (1990). The effect of xylene exposure on the liver. *Acta Morphol Hungar* 38:245-258.

[14] Ibid., p. 215, citing: Casazza JP, Felver ME, and Veech RL. (1984). The metabolism of acetone in the rat. *J Biol Chem* 259:231-236.

[15] Levin, Buck, Environmental Nutrition, p. 215, citing: Albores A, Sinal CJ, Cherian MG et al. (1995). Selective increase of rat lung cytochrome P450 1A1 dependent monooxygenase activity after acute sodium arsenite administration. *Can J Physiol Pharmocol* 73(1):153-158.

[16] Levin, Buck, Environmental Nutrition, p. 215, citing: Keyon EM, Kraichely RE, Hudson KT, it al. (1996). Differences in rates of benzene metabolism correlate with observed genotoxicity. *Toxicol Appl Pharmacol* 136(1):49-56.

[17] Levin, Buck, Environmental Nutrition, p. 215, citing: Zheng J and Hanzlik RP. (1992). Bromo(monohydroxyl)phenyl mercapturic acids: a new class of merapturic acids from bromobenzene-treated rats. *Drug Metabol Dispos* 20:688-694.

[18] Levin, Buck, Environmental Nutrition, p. 215, citing: Guengerich FP and Shimada T. (1992). Human cytochrome P450 enzymes and chemical carcinogenesis. Chapter 2. In: Jeffrey EH. (Ed). Human drug metabolism from molecular biology to man. *CRC Press*, Boca Raton, pp. 5-12.

[19] Levin, Buck, Environmental Nutrition, p. 215, citing: Guengerich FP. (1994). Metabolism and genotoxicity of dihaloalkanes. *Adv Pharmacol* 27:211-236.

[20] Levin, Buck, Environmental Nutrition, p. 215, citing: Cheever KL, Cholkis JM, et-Hawari AM et al. (1990). Ethlyene dichloride: the influence of disulfiram or ethanol on oncogenicity, metabolism and DNA covalent binding in rats. *Fund Appl Toxicol* 14(2):243-261.

[21] Levin, Buck, Environmental Nutrition, p. 215, citing: Lapadula DM. (1991). Induction of cytochrome P450 isozymes by simultaneous inhalation exposure of hens to n-hexane and methyl iso-butyl ketone (MiBK). *Biochem Pharmacol* 41(6-7):877-883.

[22] Levin, Buck, Environmental Nutrition, p. 215, citing: Kocarek TA. (1991). Selective induction of cytochrome P450e by kepone (chlordecone) in primary clutures of adult rat hepatocytes, *Mol Pharmacol* 40(2):203-210.

[23] Levin, Buck, Environmental Nutrition, p. 215, citing: Stresser DM and Kupfer D. (1997). Catalytic characteristics of CYP3A4: requirement for a phenolic fuction in ortho hydroxylation of estradiol and mono-O-demethylated methoxychlor. *Biochem* 36(8):2203-2210.

[24] Levin, Buck, Environmental Nutrition, p. 215, citing: Vezina M,

Kobusch AB, du Souich P et al. (1990). Potentiation of chloroform induced hepatotoxicity by metyl isobuty ketone and two metabolites. *Can J Physiol Pharmacol* 68(8):1055-1061.

[25] Levin, Buck, Environmental Nutrition, p. 215, citing: Hogan GK, Smith RG, and Cornish HH. (1976). Studies on the microsomal conversion of dichloromethane to carbon monoxide. *Toxicol App Pharmacol* 37:112-119.

[26] Levin, Buck, Environmental Nutrition, p. 214, citing: Levin W et al. (1982). Oxidative metabolism of polycyclic aromatic hydrocarbons to ultimate carcinogens. *Drug Metab Rev* 13:555-580.

[27] Winter, Poisons in Your Food, p. 5, citing: Howard J. Sanders, "Food Additives," *Chemical and Engineering News,* October 17, 1966. James L. Goddard, M.S., FDA Commissioner, tape-recorded interview with author, May, 1968.

[28] Winter, Ruth, Poisons in Your Food, (Crown Pub., New York, 1969) p. 5, citing: Pharmaceutical Manufacturers Association, Washington, D.C., fact booklet, 1967.

[29] Cousens, Gabriel, M.D., Rainbow Green Live-Food Cuisine, (North Atlantic Books, Berkley, CA.), p. xiv.

[30] Rogers, Sherry, M.D., Pain Free in 6 Weeks, (Prestige Publishing, Syracuse, N.Y., 2001), p. 316.

[31] Baroody, Theodore, N.D., D.C., Ph.D., Alkalize or Die Superior Health Through Proper Alkaline-Acid Balance (Holographic Health Press, Waynesville, N.C.), 2001, p. 15, 22.

[32] Young, Robert, PhD., D.Sc., Sick and Tired Reclaim Your Inner Terrain, (Woodland Publishing, Pleasant Grove, UT, 2001), p. 63-64.

[33] Young, Robert, PhD., Sick and Tired, p. 51, 61.

[34] Gruben, Rozalind, Prof., "Fasting and Detox Programmes", *Get Fresh!*, Ely, Cambridgeshire, UK, vol 2,
issue 3, Jan-Mar. 2004.

[35] Gruben, Rozalind, "Fasting and Detox Programmes," *Get Fresh!*, Jan-Mar. 2004.

[36] Gruben, Rozalind, "Fasting and Detox Programmes," *Get Fresh!*, Jan-Mar. 2004.

[37] Norman W. Walker, Raw Vegetable Juices, (Norwalk Press, Prescott, AZ), 1995 (1940).

[38] Bragg, Paul C. N.D., PhD., The Miracle of Fasting, (Health Science, Santa Barbara, CA.), 1985, p. 61.

[39] Bragg, The Miracle of Fasting, p. 57.

[40] Page, Linda, N.D., Ph.D., Detoxification, (Healthy Healing Publications, Carmel Valley, CA.), 1999, p. 63.

[41] Page, Linda, N.D., Ph.D., Detoxification, p. 18.

[42] Airola, Paavo N.D., PhD., Juice Fasting, (Health Publishers, Phoenix, Arizona), 1971, p. 40.

[43] Airola, Juice Fasting, p. 39.

[44] Airola, Juice Fasting, p. 40.

45 Airola, Juice Fasting, p. 38.
46 Walker, Norman, D.Sc., Become Younger, (Norwalk Press, Prescott, AZ), 1949, p. 11.
47 Robbins, Joel, D.C., M.D., Juicing for Health, (Health Dynamics, Tulsa, OK), p. 13, 14.
48 Bragg, The Miracle of Fasting, p. 57.
49 Airola, Paavo N.D., PhD., Juice Fasting, (Health Publishers, Phoenix, Arizona), 1971, p. 48.
50 Airola, Juice Fasting, p. 63.
51 Airola, Juice Fasting, p. 64.
52 Meyerowitz, Steve, Juice Fasting and Detoxification, (Book Pub. Company, Summertown, TN), 1999, p.14.
53 Bragg, The Miracle of Fasting, p. 86.
54 Airola, Juice Fasting, p. 49; Bragg, ibid., p. 59.
55 Airola, Juice Fasting, p. 47.
56 Airola, Juice Fasting, p. 48.
57 Bragg, Paul C. N.D., PhD., The Miracle of Fasting, (Health Science, Santa Barbara, CA.), 1985. p. 75.
58 Buchinger, Otto H.F., M.D., About Fasting a Royal Road to Healing, (Thorsons Publishers Ltd., Wellingborough, Northamptonshire), 1961, 1983, p. 62.
59 Cott, Allan, M.D., Fasting: The Ultimate Diet, (Bantam Books, NY, N.Y.), 1976, 1980, p. 97.
60 Shelton, Herbert M., Fasting for Renewal of Life, (Natural Hygiene Press, Chicago, Illinois) 1978), p. 161.
61 Shelton, Herbert M., Fasting for Renewal of Life, p. 162.
62 Hazzard, Linda Burfield, D.O., Scientific Fasting, the Ancient and Modern Key to Health, (Health Research, Mokelumne Hill, CA.), 1963, p. 183-4.
63 Lawlor, T., M.B.,B.S., and D. G. Wells, M.B., B.S., "Metabolic Hazards of Fasting", The American Journal of Clinical Nutrition., Vol. 22, No. 8, August 1969, p. 1148.
64 Lawlor, and D. G. Wells, "Metabolic Hazards of Fasting," p. 1145; (1.) Bloom, W.L. , "Fasting as an Introduction to the treatment of obesity," Metab. Clin. Exptl. 8:214, 1959. (2.) Drenick, E.J., M.E. Swendseid, W.H. Bland and S.G. Tuttle, "Prolonged starvation as treatment for severe obesity". J. Am. Med. Assoc. 187: 100, 1964. (3.) Thomson, T. J., J. Runcie and V. Miller, "Treatment of Obesity by total fasting for up to 249 days."
Lancet 2:992, 1966.
65 Lawlor, and D. G. Wells, "Metabolic Hazards of Fasting," p.1142-1145.
66 Airola, Juice Fasting, p. 34.
67 Shelton, Herbert; Oswald, Jean, Fasting for the Health of It, (Nationwide Press, Pueblo, Colorado, 1983).
68 Shelton, Herbert; Oswald, Jean, Fasting for the Health of It,

(Nationwide Press, Pueblo, Colorado, 1983).
[69]   Shelton, and Oswald, <u>Fasting for the Health of It</u>, p. 212, citing: Dr. Benesh and Dr. McEachen.
[70]   Shelton, and Oswald, <u>Fasting for the Health of It</u>, p. 211, citing: Dr. William Esser.
[71]   Shelton, and Oswald, <u>Fasting for the Health of It</u>, p. 213, citing: Dr. Robert Gross.
[72]   Young, Robert, O., a research scientist at pH Miracle Living Center, citing study on his website 11/2007.
[73]   Airola, Paavo, PhD, ND, <u>Cancer Causes, Prevention and Treatment, the Total Approach,</u> (Health Plus, Publishers, Sherwood, Oregon, 97140, 1972), pp. 9, 28, 34.
[74]   Airola, Paavo, PhD, ND, <u>Cancer Causes, Prevention and Treatment, the Total Approach,</u> pp. 9, 28, 34.   Airola, Paavo O., <u>How to Get Well,</u> (Health Plus Publishers, P.O. Box 1027, Sherwood, Oregon, 97140).
[75]   Red Beet Juice therapy for cancer and leukemia, as recommended by Dr. Siegmund Schmidt and Dr. A. Ferenezi - *March of Truth on Cancer*, (Arlin Brown Inf. Center, P.O. Box 251, Fort Belvoir, Virgina, 22060).
[76]   "Modified Grape Cure" and "<u>Grape Cure</u>". (Arlin Brown Inf. Center, P.O. Box 251, Fort Belvoir, Virginia, 22060).
[77]   Airola, Paavo O., <u>Are You Confused?</u>, (Health Plus Pub., P.O. Box 1027, Sherwood, Oregon, 97140).
[78]   Breuss Vegetable Juice, a product of Switzerland, distributed by CAJ Food Products, Inc.
[79]   Breuss, Rudolf, <u>The Breuss Cancer Cure</u>, (Alive Books, Burnaby BC Canada, 1995), p. 28-29.
[80]   Breuss, Rudolf, <u>The Breuss Cancer Cure</u>, p. 33.
[81]   Rancout, J., <u>Lac Simon</u>, Quebec, March 27, 1995.
[82]   Breuss, Rudolf, <u>The Breuss Cancer Cure</u>, Forward, p. ix-x.
[83]   Airola, Paavo N.D., PhD., <u>Juice Fasting</u>, (Health Publishers, Phoenix, Arizona), 1971), p. 42.
[84]   Bragg, Paul, N.D., PhD., <u>The Miracle of Fasting</u>, (Health Science, Santa Barbara, CA., 1985), p. 82
[85]   Bragg, Paul, <u>The Miracle of Fasting</u>, p. 67.
[86]   Walker, Norman, W., M.D., D.Sc., <u>Diet and Salad</u>, (Norwalk Press, Prescott, AZ), 1995 (1940), p. 3.
[87]   Walker, Norman, <u>Diet and Salad</u>, p. 87, 90 .
[88]   Walker, Norman, <u>Colon Health, The Key to Vibrant Life</u>, (Norwalk Press, Prescott, AZ, 1995), p. 11.
[89]   Walker, Norman, <u>Colon Health, The Key to Vibrant Life</u>, p. 13.
[90]   Jensen, Bernard, D.C., Ph.D., <u>Dr. Jensen's Guide to Better Bowel Care</u>, (Avery Pub., N.Y., N.Y., 1999), p. 10.
[91]   Jensen, Bernard, <u>Dr. Jensen's Guide to Better Bowel Care</u>, p. 19.

[92] Jensen, Bernard, <u>Dr. Jensen's Guide to Better Bowel Care</u>, p. 20.

[93] Weinberger, Stanley, C.M.T., <u>Healing Within: The Complete Guide to Colon Health, Healing</u> (Within Products, Larkspur, CA), p. 39, 43.

[94] Weinberger, Stanley, <u>Parasites an Epidemic in Disguise</u>, (Healing Within Products, Larkspur, CA, 1993), p. 1, 3.

[95] Weinberger, Stanley, <u>Parasites an Epidemic in Disguise</u>, from: *The Miami Herald*, Dolly Kaltz, June 25, 1978.

[96] Weinberger, Stanley, <u>Parasites an Epidemic in Disguise</u>, p. 9; reprinted from the *Chicago Tribune* Service, Ronald Kotulak.

[97] Weinberger, Stanley, <u>Parasites an Epidemic in Disguise</u>, p. 15, 21.

[98] Weinberger, Stanley, <u>Healling Within,</u> p. 81.

[99] Hanna Kroeger MsD, <u>Parasites The Enemy Within</u>, (Bolder, Colorado), 1991, p. 2, 55.

[100] Clark, Hulda Regehr, Ph.D., N.D. , <u>The Cure for All Diseases</u>, (New Century Press, San Diego, CA), 1995, p. 2.

[101] Clark, Hulda Regehr, <u>The Cure for All Diseases</u>, p. 33.

[102] Clark, Hulda Regehr, <u>The Cure for All Diseases</u>, p. 97.

[103] <u>Gerson Therapy Handbook</u>, *A Coffee Enema? Now I've Heard Everything*, Gar Hildenbrand, p. 75, citing: Gerson Healing Newsletter #13, May-June 1989.

[104] Gerson, M. 1979, *Physiological Chemistry and Physics*, 1095); 449-464, 1978. "The Cure of Advanced Cancer by Diet Therapy, a Summary of 30 Years of Clinical Experimentation."

[105] <u>Gerson Therapy Handbook</u>, *A Coffee Enema?,* p. 77.

[106] Airola, Paavo, <u>Juice Fasting</u>, p. 66.

[107] Airola, Paavo, <u>Juice Fasting</u>, p. 67.

[108] Shelton, Herbert, M., N.D., Oswald, Jean A., <u>Fasting for the Health of It</u>, (Nationwide Press, Ltd., P.O. Box 1528, Pueblo, Colorado, 81002), 1983, p. 147.

[109] Willis, Pauline, <u>The Reflexology Manual</u>, (Healing Arts Press, One Park Street, Rochester, Vermont 05767, 1995), p. 11.

[110] Bragg, Paul, <u>The Miracle of Fasting</u>, p. 84.

[111] Adventist Health Study-2, Loma Linda University, Loma Linda, CA.

[112] Horne, Ross, <u>Improving on Pritikin</u>, (Happy Landings Pty Ltd., P.O. Box 277 Avalon Beach, N.S.W. Australia, 1989), p. 197.

[113] Airola, Paavo, Ph.D., N.D., <u>Rejuvenation Secrets from around the World</u>, (Health plus Pub., Phoenix, AZ, 1974), (*Nutrition Today*, Vol. 8, Number 5, October /November, 1973.)

[114] Airola, Paavo, <u>Rejuvenation Secrets ...</u>, p. 113-114.

[115] Airola, Paavo, <u>Rejuvenation Secrets ...</u>, p. 61-62.

[116] Airola, Paavo, <u>Rejuvenation Secrets ...</u>, p. 113-114.

[117] Airola, Paavo, <u>Rejuvenation Secrets ...</u>, p. 62.

[118] AThe Seventh Day Adventist: Why do They Live Longer?@ *Health Quarterly*, (Nov/Dec 1981).

[119] Robert Cohen, *Milk A-Z*, (Argus Publishing, 325 Sylvan Ave., Englewood Cliffs, NJ, 07632, 2001), p. 52, citing: *Journal of the*

American Dietetic Association, November 1997, 97(1).

[120]   Robert Cohen, *Milk A-Z*, page 52, citing: *British Medical Journal*, 1996; 313.

[121]   Lee, C., et al. AAge Associated Alterations of the Mitochondrial Genome,@ *Free Rad Bio Med* 22, 7 (1977): 1259-69. Quoted from Peter Bennett, N.D., Stephen Barrie, N.D., 7-Day Detox Miracle, (Prima Health, Roseville, CA.), 1999, p. 255.

[122]   John Gainer, "Now the Villain is Protein," *Science News* (August 21, 1971): 123-24.

[123]   Wolfe, David; *Eating for Beauty,* p. 206.

[124]   Adams JS, Clemens TL, Parrish JA, Holick MF. Vitamin D Synthesis and metabolism after ultraviolet irradiation of normal and vitamin D deficient subjects. *N Engl J Med* 1982, Mar 25;306(12):722-5.

[125]   Adams JS, Clemens TL, Parrish JA, Holick MF. Vitamin D Synthesis and metabolism after ultraviolet irradiation of normal and vitamin D deficient subjects. *N Engl J Med* 1982, Mar 25;306(12):722-5.

[126]   Adams JS, Clemens TL, Parrish JA, Holick MF. Vitamin D Synthesis and metabolism after ultraviolet irradiation of normal and vitamin D deficient subjects. *N Engl J Med* 1982, Mar 25;306(12):722-5.

[127]   Adams JS, Clemens TL, Parrish JA, Holick MF. Vitamin D Synthesis and metabolism after ultraviolet irradiation of normal and vitamin D deficient subjects. *N Engl J Med* 1982, Mar 25,306(12):722-5.

[128]   Salloum, Trevor K., N.D., Fasting Signs and Symptoms A Clinical Guide, (Buckeye Naturopathic Press, East Palestine, Ohio, 1992), citing: Sheldon HM. The Science and fine art of fasting. Chicago: Natural Hygiene Press; 1978.

[129]   "The Seventh Day Adventist: Why do They Live Longer?" *Health Quarterly*, (Nov/Dec 1981).

[130]   Malkmus, *God's Way...*, p. 135; the *Diamonds in Living Health*.

[131]   Baker, Elizabeth, *The Gourmet Uncook Book, The Elegance of Raw Foods*, Promotion Publishing, San Diego, CA.. 1996, p. 23-24.

[132]   Graham, Douglas, Dr., *The High Energy Diet Recipe Guide*, The Cause of Health, Marathon, FL, p. xii, xiii.

[133]   Farrell, Walter, O.P., *My Way of Life Pocket Edition of St. Thomas the Summa Simplified for Everyone*, (Confraternity of the Precious Blood, BroOklyn, NY, 1952), p. 280, 281.

[134]   Campbell, Colin, *The China Study*, (Benbella books, Dallas, 2004).

[135]   Encyclopedia of the Early Church, (Institutum Patristicum Augustinianum, Oxford University Press, New York, N.Y., 1992), citing: Paed. II 1, 1-2, 34; III 12, 90.

[136]   Encyclopedia of the Early Church, citing: Cels. 5, 49 and 8, 30.

[137]   Encyclopedia of the Early Church, citing: In *Lev.* 10, 1-2; cf. Ambr., *In Ps.* 40, 1: Greg. Nyss., Beat. IV; Util. ieiun. 1,1.

[138]   Encyclopedia of the Early Church, citing: Basil, Ieiun. Hom. 2, 5; cf. Chrom., Serm. 35.4 and In Mt. 29.

[139]   Encyclopedia of the Early Church, citing: Ambr., Hel. 3,4; 4,7;

Ep 63, 17).

[140] Encyclopedia of the Early Church, citing: Athan., Ant. 7,6.

[141] Encyclopedia of the Early Church, citing: Via Pach. 25.

[142] Encyclopedia of the Early Church, citing: Jov. 2,6; Ep 54, 105.

[143] Encyclopedia of the Early Church, citing: Basil, *Ieiun.* 1 and 2; Cass., *Coll* 21.13ff, and Inst. *coen.* 5,5 ff; cf. Hipp., *Trad.* ap. 25; Epiph., *Haer.* 3; Exp. *fid.* 23; Theodor., *Haer. fab.* 5,29.

[144] Encyclopedia of the Early Church, citing: Rule 4,39-41, 49.

[145] Encyclopedia of the Early Church, citing: 12-20; 39-50; 86-94, *Serm.* 13,1.

[146] St. Francis of Assisi, Omnibus of Sources, (Franciscan Herald Press, Chicago, Illinois), 1983, p. 34.

[147] Vanzillotta, Gino, O.M., books: The Third Order of Minims (Los Angeles, CA., 2001); Francis the "Minim" (Los Angeles, CA., 2001); Life of St. Francis of Paola, translation, written by: Anonymous Disciple Contemporary with the Saint (Los Angeles, CA., 2002).

www.ingramcontent.com/pod-product-compliance
Lightning Source LLC
Chambersburg PA
CBHW020436290526
45785CB00002B/873